CARB
COUNTER

Larger version of this book, with up to 6 portion photos for each food!

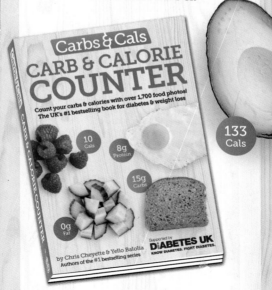

Carbs & Cals

CARB & CALORIE
COUNTER

Count your carbs & calories with over 1,700 food photos!
The UK's #1 bestselling book for diabetes & weight loss

10 Cals

8g Protein

15g Carbs

0g Fat

133 Cals

by Chris Cheyette & Yello Balolia
Authors of the #1 bestselling series

Supported by
DIABETES UK
KNOW DIABETES. FIGHT DIABETES.

Carbs & Cals
POCKET COUNTER

3RD EDITION

First published in Great Britain in 2011
3rd edition published in 2016

by Chello Publishing Limited
Registered Company Number 7237986
Copyright © Chello Publishing Limited 2016

www.chellopublishing.co.uk
info@chellopublishing.co.uk

This edition is in association with Diabetes UK. Diabetes UK
is the operating name of The British Diabetic Association.
Company limited by guarantee. Registered in England
Number 339181. Registered office: Macleod House, 10
Parkway, London NW1 7AA. A charity registered in England
and Wales (215199) and in Scotland (SC039136).

ISBN: 978-1-908261-19-9   Printed in Malta 0818

Carbs & Cals was written by:
Chris Cheyette BSc (Hons) MSc RD, Diabetes Dietitian
and Yello Balolia BA (Hons).

For more information, please visit:
www.carbsandcals.com

Foreword

Carbs & Cals is a great tool for those people with diabetes who count carbohydrates as part of the management of their condition. This easy-to-use visual reference guide allows you to compare what is on your plate with the pictures in the book, to find out the amount of carbohydrate and calories in the food you are eating.

Whatever your goals, we are sure that you will find Carbs & Cals a great help in achieving them.

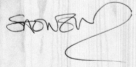

Simon O'Neill
Director of Health Intelligence
and Professional Liaison
Diabetes UK

DiABETES UK
KNOW DIABETES. FIGHT DIABETES.

www.diabetes.org.uk

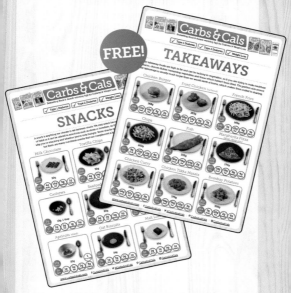

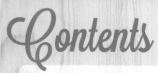
Contents

Introduction

Welcome to the Carbs & Cals POCKET COUNTER. This condensed book contains over 800 photos of a wide range of popular food and drink items. The carb, calorie, protein, fat, saturated fat and fibre values are clearly displayed in colour-coded circles below each photo.

This highly visual approach makes it incredibly quick and easy to see the nutrient content of the food and drink you consume.

This nifty POCKET COUNTER is the ideal support tool to carry with you at all times for healthy eating, weight management and portion control. If you have diabetes, it can also provide helpful guidance with carb counting.

For a greater variety of photos (over 1,700 in total and up to 6 portion sizes for each food), and further helpful information on nutrients, healthy eating, weight loss and diabetes management, please see the full-size version: the Carbs & Cals CARB & CALORIE COUNTER.

For more information, please visit:
www.carbsandcals.com

How to use this book

1. Decide what you want to eat or drink and find the meal, drink or snack in the book.

2. Look at the circles below the photo for the values you are interested in. These show the carbs, calories, protein, fat, sat fat, fibre and 5-a-day.

3. Choose your portion size and assemble your meal.

4. Add up the carbs, cals, protein, fat, sat fat, fibre and 5-a-day values for the different food components, to give the totals for your meal.

8g Carbs

58 Cals

1g Prot

3g Fat

2g SatFat

0g Fibre

Key points when using this book

The weight of each portion is stated below each photo, just in case you want to double check the weight of your own portion. This is always the cooked/prepared weight.

Values for carbs, protein, fat, saturated fat and fibre are given to the nearest gram. Therefore, if a food has 0.4g of fat, the value will be listed as 0g. If a food has 0.6g of fat, the value will be listed as 1g.

All foods in this book are shown on one of the following dishes. You may wish to use plates and bowls that are the same size as the ones in the book:

20cm side plate
26cm dinner plate
14cm cereal bowl
22cm large bowl

Bourbon Cream

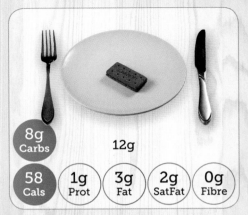

8g Carbs

12g

58 Cals | 1g Prot | 3g Fat | 2g SatFat | 0g Fibre

Chocolate Digestive

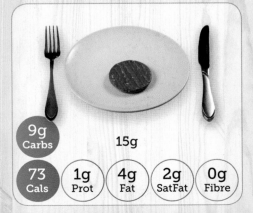

9g Carbs

15g

73 Cals | 1g Prot | 4g Fat | 2g SatFat | 0g Fibre

Chocolate Chip Cookie

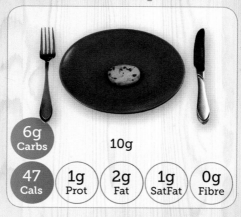

6g Carbs

10g

47 Cals | **1g** Prot | **2g** Fat | **1g** SatFat | **0g** Fibre

Chocolate Oat Biscuit

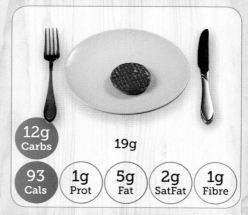

12g Carbs

19g

93 Cals | **1g** Prot | **5g** Fat | **2g** SatFat | **1g** Fibre

Chocolate Sandwich Biscuit

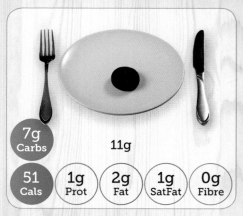

7g Carbs

11g

51 Cals | 1g Prot | 2g Fat | 1g SatFat | 0g Fibre

Custard Cream

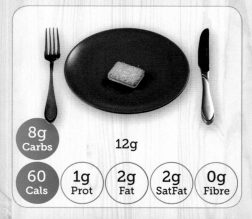

8g Carbs

12g

60 Cals | 1g Prot | 2g Fat | 2g SatFat | 0g Fibre

Digestive

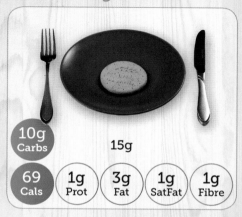

10g Carbs

15g

69 Cals | **1g** Prot | **3g** Fat | **1g** SatFat | **1g** Fibre

Fig Roll

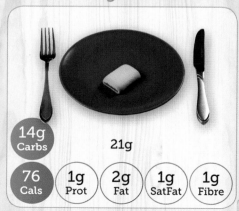

14g Carbs

21g

76 Cals | **1g** Prot | **2g** Fat | **1g** SatFat | **1g** Fibre

Ginger Biscuit

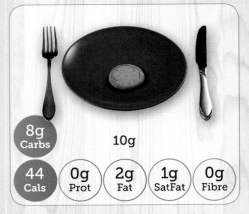

8g Carbs

10g

44 Cals | **0g** Prot | **2g** Fat | **1g** SatFat | **0g** Fibre

Gingerbread Man

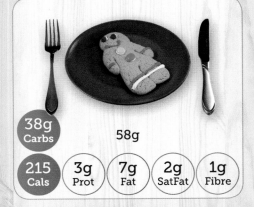

38g Carbs

58g

215 Cals | **3g** Prot | **7g** Fat | **2g** SatFat | **1g** Fibre

Iced Ring

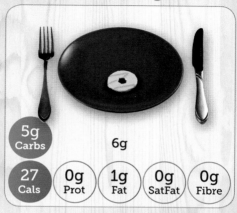

5g Carbs

6g

27 Cals

0g Prot

1g Fat

0g SatFat

0g Fibre

Jaffa Cake

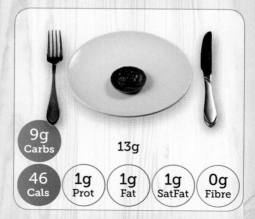

9g Carbs

13g

46 Cals

1g Prot

1g Fat

1g SatFat

0g Fibre

Jam Ring

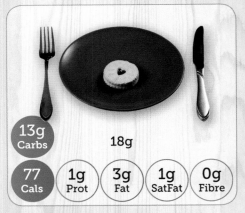

13g Carbs

18g

77 Cals

1g Prot

3g Fat

1g SatFat

0g Fibre

Malted Milk

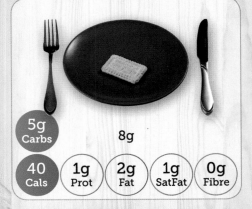

5g Carbs

8g

40 Cals

1g Prot

2g Fat

1g SatFat

0g Fibre

Milk Chocolate Biscuit Bar

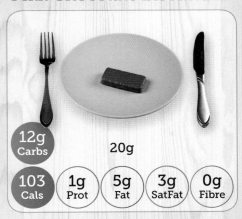

12g Carbs

20g

103 Cals

1g Prot

5g Fat

3g SatFat

0g Fibre

Milk Chocolate Finger

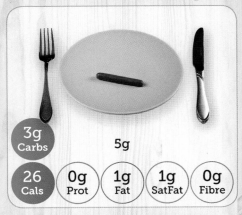

3g Carbs

5g

26 Cals

0g Prot

1g Fat

1g SatFat

0g Fibre

Milk Chocolate Wafer

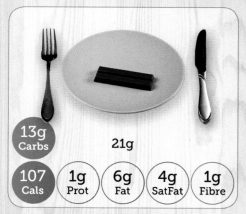

13g Carbs

21g

107 Cals

1g Prot

6g Fat

4g SatFat

1g Fibre

Nice Biscuit

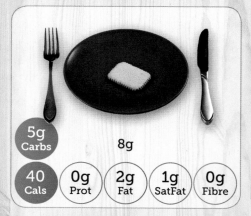

5g Carbs

8g

40 Cals

0g Prot

2g Fat

1g SatFat

0g Fibre

Oat Biscuit

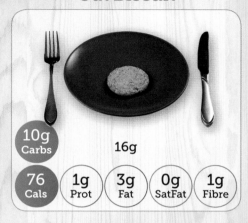

10g Carbs

16g

76 Cals | 1g Prot | 3g Fat | 0g SatFat | 1g Fibre

Pink Wafer

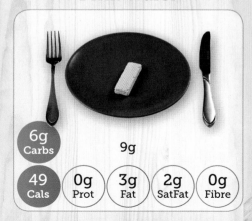

6g Carbs

9g

49 Cals | 0g Prot | 3g Fat | 2g SatFat | 0g Fibre

Rich Tea

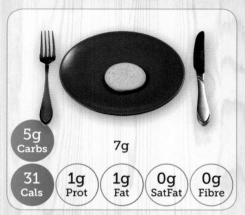

5g Carbs

7g

31 Cals

1g Prot

1g Fat

0g SatFat

0g Fibre

Shortbread Finger

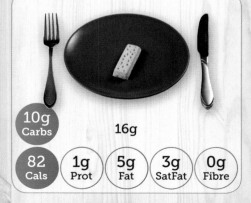

10g Carbs

16g

82 Cals

1g Prot

5g Fat

3g SatFat

0g Fibre

Shortcake

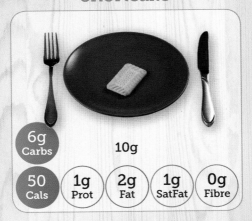

6g Carbs

10g

50 Cals

1g Prot

2g Fat

1g SatFat

0g Fibre

Breadstick

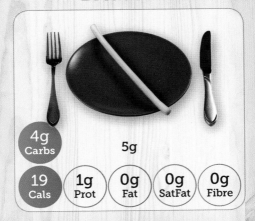

4g Carbs

5g

19 Cals

1g Prot

0g Fat

0g SatFat

0g Fibre

Cheddar

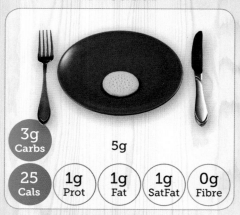

3g Carbs

5g

25 Cals | **1g** Prot | **1g** Fat | **1g** SatFat | **0g** Fibre

Cheese Straw

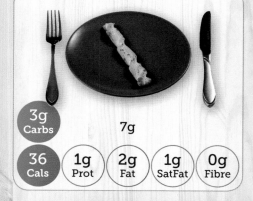

3g Carbs

7g

36 Cals | **1g** Prot | **2g** Fat | **1g** SatFat | **0g** Fibre

Cream Cracker

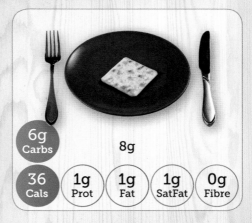

6g Carbs

8g

36 Cals | 1g Prot | 1g Fat | 1g SatFat | 0g Fibre

Crispbread

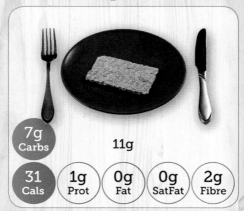

7g Carbs

11g

31 Cals | 1g Prot | 0g Fat | 0g SatFat | 2g Fibre

Digestive (savoury)

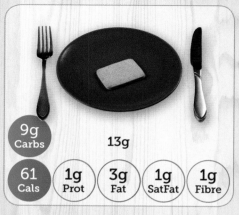

9g Carbs

13g

61 Cals

1g Prot

3g Fat

1g SatFat

1g Fibre

Oatcake

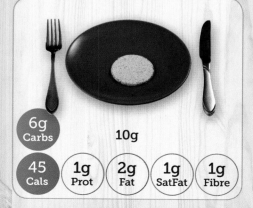

6g Carbs

10g

45 Cals

1g Prot

2g Fat

1g SatFat

1g Fibre

Puffed Cracker

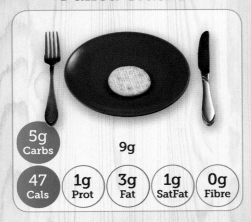

5g Carbs

9g

47 Cals

1g Prot

3g Fat

1g SatFat

0g Fibre

Rice Cake

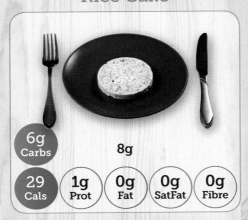

6g Carbs

8g

29 Cals

1g Prot

0g Fat

0g SatFat

0g Fibre

Water Biscuit

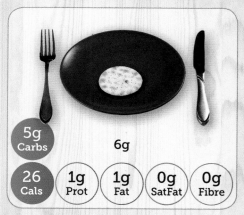

5g Carbs

6g

26 Cals | **1g** Prot | **1g** Fat | **0g** SatFat | **0g** Fibre

Wholegrain Cracker

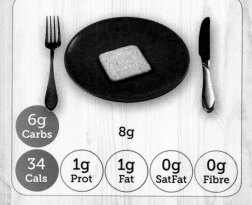

6g Carbs

8g

34 Cals | **1g** Prot | **1g** Fat | **0g** SatFat | **0g** Fibre

Granary Bread

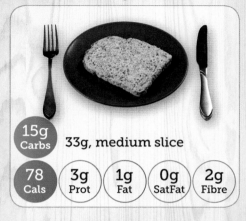

15g Carbs
33g, medium slice

78 Cals | **3g** Prot | **1g** Fat | **0g** SatFat | **2g** Fibre

White Bread

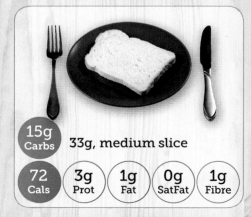

15g Carbs
33g, medium slice

72 Cals | **3g** Prot | **1g** Fat | **0g** SatFat | **1g** Fibre

Wholemeal Bread

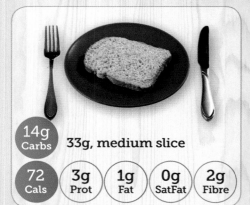

14g Carbs

33g, medium slice

72 Cals | **3g** Prot | **1g** Fat | **0g** SatFat | **2g** Fibre

White Wholemeal Bread

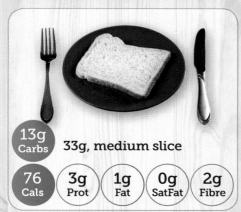

13g Carbs

33g, medium slice

76 Cals | **3g** Prot | **1g** Fat | **0g** SatFat | **2g** Fibre

Bap (white)

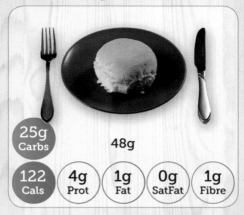

25g Carbs

48g

122 Cals | **4g** Prot | **1g** Fat | **0g** SatFat | **1g** Fibre

Bap (wholemeal)

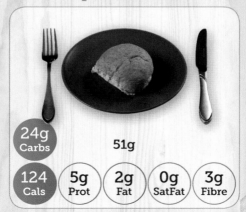

24g Carbs

51g

124 Cals | **5g** Prot | **2g** Fat | **0g** SatFat | **3g** Fibre

Crusty Roll (white)

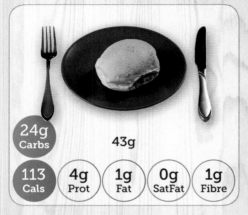

24g Carbs

43g

113 Cals

4g Prot

1g Fat

0g SatFat

1g Fibre

Bagel

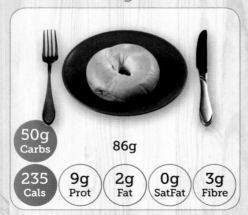

50g Carbs

86g

235 Cals

9g Prot

2g Fat

0g SatFat

3g Fibre

English Muffin

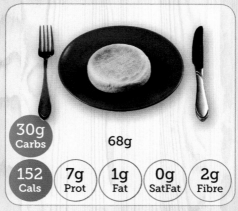

30g Carbs

68g

152 Cals | **7g** Prot | **1g** Fat | **0g** SatFat | **2g** Fibre

Crumpet

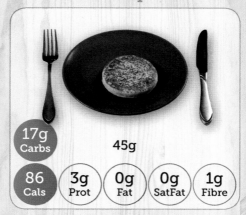

17g Carbs

45g

86 Cals | **3g** Prot | **0g** Fat | **0g** SatFat | **1g** Fibre

Poppy Seeded Roll

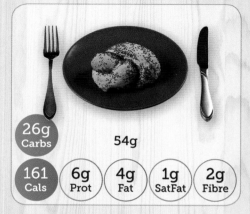

26g Carbs

54g

161 Cals

6g Prot

4g Fat

1g SatFat

2g Fibre

Tea Cake

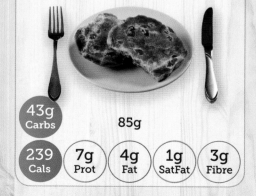

43g Carbs

85g

239 Cals

7g Prot

4g Fat

1g SatFat

3g Fibre

Burger Bun

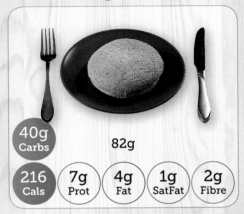

40g Carbs

82g

216 Cals

7g Prot

4g Fat

1g SatFat

2g Fibre

Finger Roll

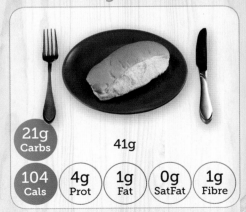

21g Carbs

41g

104 Cals

4g Prot

1g Fat

0g SatFat

1g Fibre

Croutons

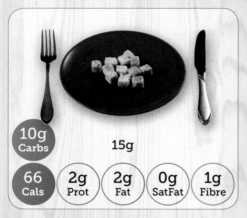

10g Carbs

15g

66 Cals

2g Prot

2g Fat

0g SatFat

1g Fibre

Ciabatta

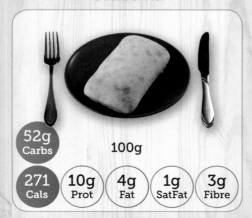

52g Carbs

100g

271 Cals

10g Prot

4g Fat

1g SatFat

3g Fibre

Panini

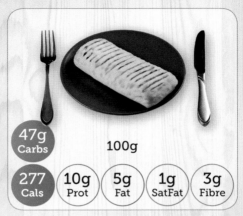

47g Carbs

100g

277 Cals

10g Prot

5g Fat

1g SatFat

3g Fibre

Baguette

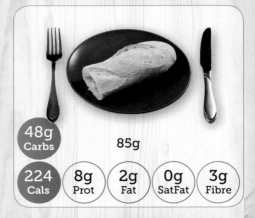

48g Carbs

85g

224 Cals

8g Prot

2g Fat

0g SatFat

3g Fibre

Banana Bread

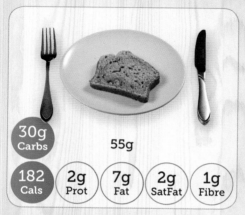

30g Carbs

55g

182 Cals

2g Prot

7g Fat

2g SatFat

1g Fibre

Focaccia

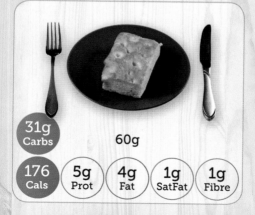

31g Carbs

60g

176 Cals

5g Prot

4g Fat

1g SatFat

1g Fibre

Garlic Bread

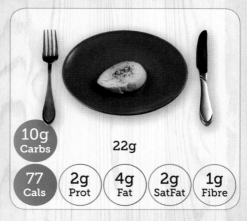

10g Carbs

22g

77 Cals | 2g Prot | 4g Fat | 2g SatFat | 1g Fibre

Pumpernickel

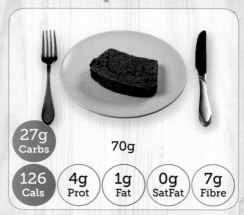

27g Carbs

70g

126 Cals | 4g Prot | 1g Fat | 0g SatFat | 7g Fibre

Raisin Bread

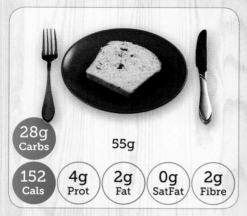

28g Carbs

55g

152 Cals

4g Prot

2g Fat

0g SatFat

2g Fibre

Rye Bread

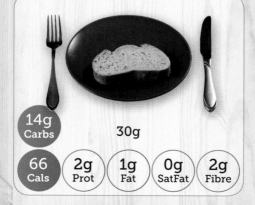

14g Carbs

30g

66 Cals

2g Prot

1g Fat

0g SatFat

2g Fibre

Sourdough

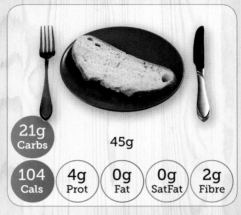

21g Carbs

45g

104 Cals

4g Prot

0g Fat

0g SatFat

2g Fibre

Spelt Bread

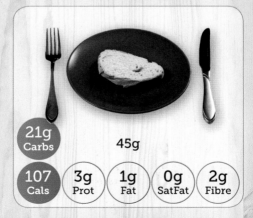

21g Carbs

45g

107 Cals

3g Prot

1g Fat

0g SatFat

2g Fibre

Pitta Bread (white)

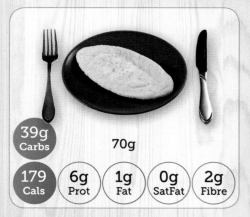

39g Carbs

70g

179 Cals | **6g** Prot | **1g** Fat | **0g** SatFat | **2g** Fibre

Pitta Bread (wholemeal)

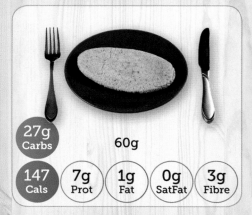

27g Carbs

60g

147 Cals | **7g** Prot | **1g** Fat | **0g** SatFat | **3g** Fibre

Turkish Flatbread

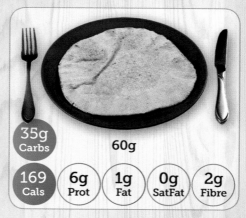

35g Carbs

60g

169 Cals | 6g Prot | 1g Fat | 0g SatFat | 2g Fibre

Taco Shell

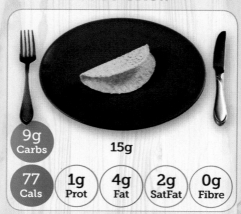

9g Carbs

15g

77 Cals | 1g Prot | 4g Fat | 2g SatFat | 0g Fibre

Tortilla (flour)

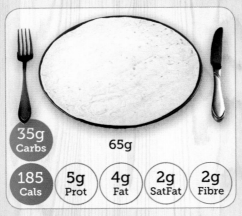

65g

35g Carbs

185 Cals | **5g** Prot | **4g** Fat | **2g** SatFat | **2g** Fibre

Naan Bread

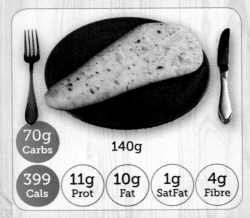

140g

70g Carbs

399 Cals | **11g** Prot | **10g** Fat | **1g** SatFat | **4g** Fibre

Poppadom

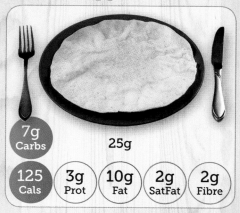

7g Carbs

25g

125 Cals

3g Prot

10g Fat

2g SatFat

2g Fibre

Paratha

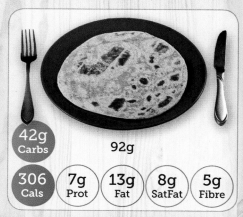

42g Carbs

92g

306 Cals

7g Prot

13g Fat

8g SatFat

5g Fibre

Chapati (without fat)

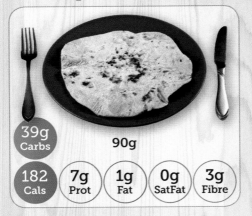

39g Carbs

90g

182 Cals | **7g** Prot | **1g** Fat | **0g** SatFat | **3g** Fibre

Chapati (with butter)

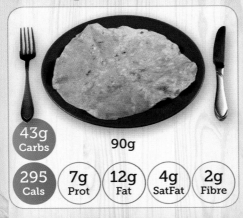

43g Carbs

90g

295 Cals | **7g** Prot | **12g** Fat | **4g** SatFat | **2g** Fibre

Puri

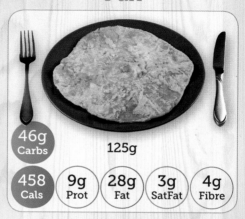

46g
Carbs

125g

458
Cals

9g
Prot

28g
Fat

3g
SatFat

4g
Fibre

Roti

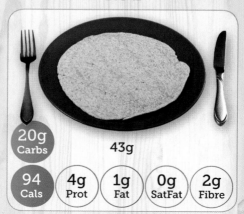

20g
Carbs

43g

94
Cals

4g
Prot

1g
Fat

0g
SatFat

2g
Fibre

Brioche

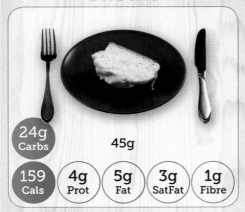

24g Carbs

45g

159 Cals | **4g** Prot | **5g** Fat | **3g** SatFat | **1g** Fibre

Croissant

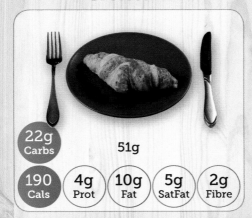

22g Carbs

51g

190 Cals | **4g** Prot | **10g** Fat | **5g** SatFat | **2g** Fibre

Pain au Chocolat

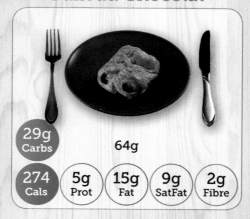

29g Carbs

64g

274 Cals

5g Prot

15g Fat

9g SatFat

2g Fibre

All Bran

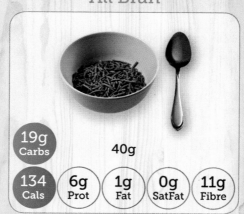

19g Carbs

40g

134 Cals

6g Prot

1g Fat

0g SatFat

11g Fibre

Bran Flakes

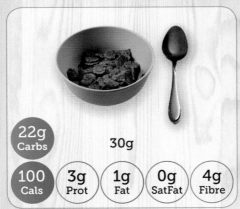

22g Carbs

30g

100 Cals | **3g** Prot | **1g** Fat | **0g** SatFat | **4g** Fibre

Chocolate Snaps

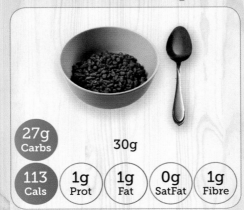

27g Carbs

30g

113 Cals | **1g** Prot | **1g** Fat | **0g** SatFat | **1g** Fibre

Corn Flakes

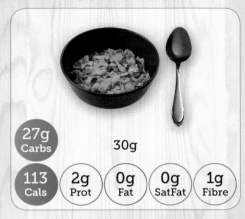

27g Carbs

30g

113 Cals

2g Prot

0g Fat

0g SatFat

1g Fibre

Frosted Flakes

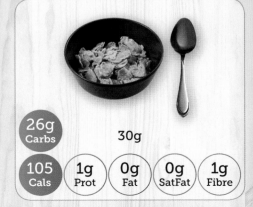

26g Carbs

30g

105 Cals

1g Prot

0g Fat

0g SatFat

1g Fibre

Fruit & Fibre

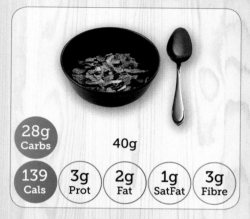

28g Carbs

40g

139 Cals

3g Prot

2g Fat

1g SatFat

3g Fibre

Granola

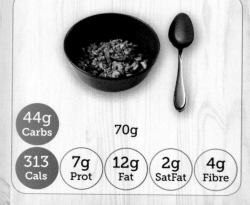

44g Carbs

70g

313 Cals

7g Prot

12g Fat

2g SatFat

4g Fibre

Honey Nut Flakes

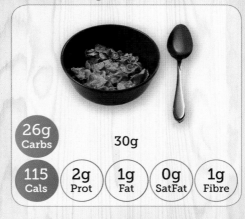

26g Carbs

30g

115 Cals | **2g** Prot | **1g** Fat | **0g** SatFat | **1g** Fibre

Honey Puffed Wheat

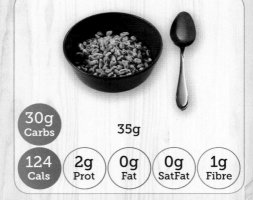

30g Carbs

35g

124 Cals | **2g** Prot | **0g** Fat | **0g** SatFat | **1g** Fibre

Malted Wheats

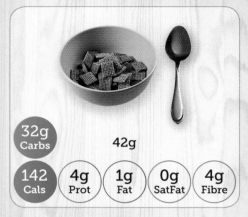

32g Carbs

42g

142 Cals

4g Prot

1g Fat

0g SatFat

4g Fibre

Muesli

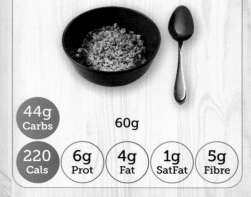

44g Carbs

60g

220 Cals

6g Prot

4g Fat

1g SatFat

5g Fibre

Multigrain Hoops

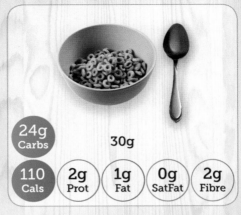

24g Carbs

30g

110 Cals

2g Prot

1g Fat

0g SatFat

2g Fibre

Raisin Bites

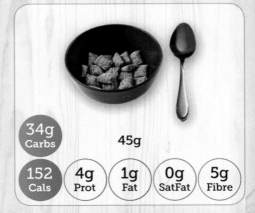

34g Carbs

45g

152 Cals

4g Prot

1g Fat

0g SatFat

5g Fibre

Rice Snaps

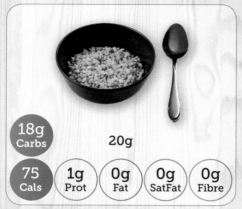

18g Carbs

20g

75 Cals

1g Prot

0g Fat

0g SatFat

0g Fibre

Special Flakes with Berries

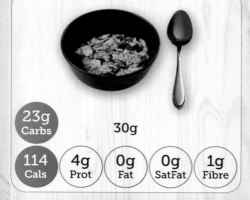

23g Carbs

30g

114 Cals

4g Prot

0g Fat

0g SatFat

1g Fibre

Oat Biscuit

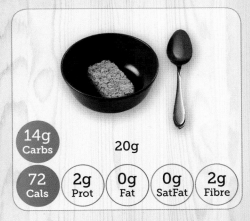

14g
Carbs

20g

72
Cals

2g
Prot

0g
Fat

0g
SatFat

2g
Fibre

Wheat Biscuit

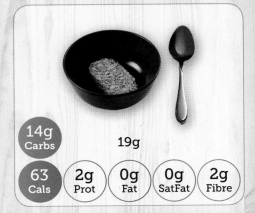

14g
Carbs

19g

63
Cals

2g
Prot

0g
Fat

0g
SatFat

2g
Fibre

Wheat Pillow

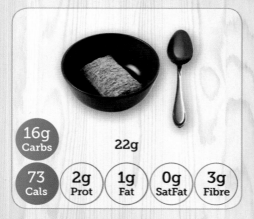

16g Carbs

22g

73 Cals · **2g** Prot · **1g** Fat · **0g** SatFat · **3g** Fibre

Milk (whole)

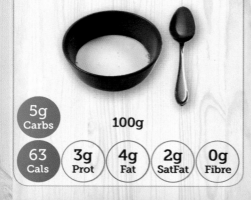

5g Carbs

100g

63 Cals · **3g** Prot · **4g** Fat · **2g** SatFat · **0g** Fibre

Milk (semi-skimmed)

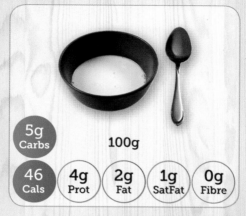

5g Carbs

100g

46 Cals · 4g Prot · 2g Fat · 1g SatFat · 0g Fibre

Milk (skimmed)

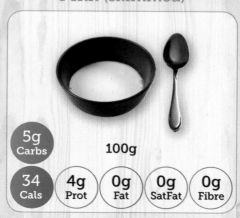

5g Carbs

100g

34 Cals · 4g Prot · 0g Fat · 0g SatFat · 0g Fibre

Cornmeal Porridge
(with condensed milk)

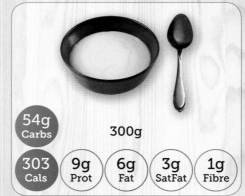

54g Carbs

303 Cals

9g Prot

6g Fat

3g SatFat

1g Fibre

300g

Cornmeal Porridge
(with water)

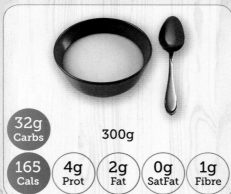

32g Carbs

165 Cals

4g Prot

2g Fat

0g SatFat

1g Fibre

300g

Porridge
(with semi-skimmed milk)

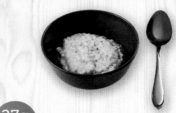

27g Carbs

220g (27g oats)

185 Cals

10g Prot

5g Fat

2g SatFat

2g Fibre

Porridge
(with water)

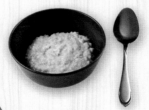

19g Carbs

220g (27g oats)

103 Cals

3g Prot

2g Fat

0g SatFat

2g Fibre

Toast with Choc Spread
& butter

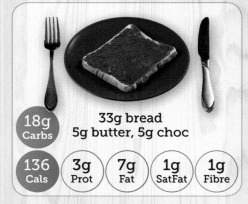

18g Carbs

33g bread
5g butter, 5g choc

136 Cals

3g Prot | **7g** Fat | **1g** SatFat | **1g** Fibre

Toast with Honey
& butter

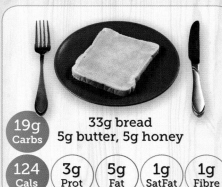

19g Carbs

33g bread
5g butter, 5g honey

124 Cals

3g Prot | **5g** Fat | **1g** SatFat | **1g** Fibre

Toast with Jam
& butter

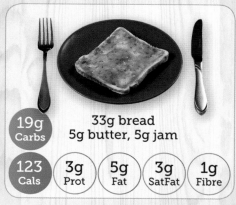

19g Carbs

33g bread
5g butter, 5g jam

123 Cals | **3g** Prot | **5g** Fat | **3g** SatFat | **1g** Fibre

Toast with Lemon Curd
& butter

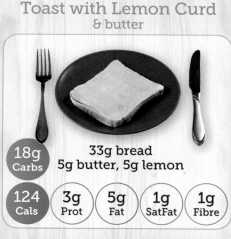

18g Carbs

33g bread
5g butter, 5g lemon

124 Cals | **3g** Prot | **5g** Fat | **1g** SatFat | **1g** Fibre

Toast with Marmalade
& butter

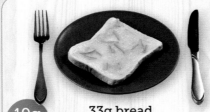

19g Carbs

33g bread
5g butter, 5g marmalade

123 Cals | **3g** Prot | **5g** Fat | **1g** SatFat | **1g** Fibre

Toast with Peanut Butter
& butter

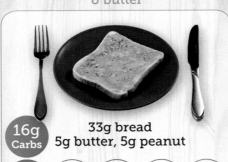

16g Carbs

33g bread
5g butter, 5g peanut

140 Cals | **4g** Prot | **7g** Fat | **3g** SatFat | **1g** Fibre

Low-carb Cooked Breakfast

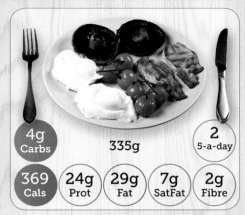

4g Carbs

335g

2 5-a-day

369 Cals | **24g** Prot | **29g** Fat | **7g** SatFat | **2g** Fibre

Kippers, Spinach & Peppers

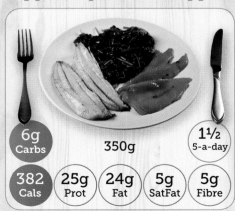

6g Carbs

350g

1½ 5-a-day

382 Cals | **25g** Prot | **24g** Fat | **5g** SatFat | **5g** Fibre

Scrambled Eggs, Tomatoes & Halloumi

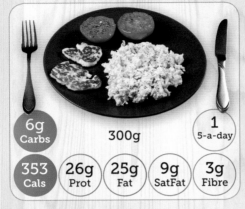

6g Carbs

300g

1 5-a-day

353 Cals

26g Prot

25g Fat

9g SatFat

3g Fibre

Pancake (plain)

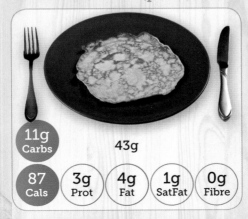

11g Carbs

43g

87 Cals

3g Prot

4g Fat

1g SatFat

0g Fibre

Pancake with Choc Spread

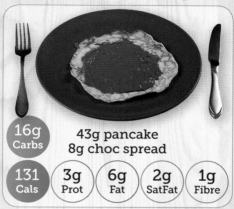

16g Carbs

43g pancake
8g choc spread

131 Cals | **3g** Prot | **6g** Fat | **2g** SatFat | **1g** Fibre

Pancake with Maple Syrup

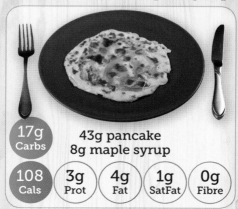

17g Carbs

43g pancake
8g maple syrup

108 Cals | **3g** Prot | **4g** Fat | **1g** SatFat | **0g** Fibre

Pancake with Sugar & Lemon

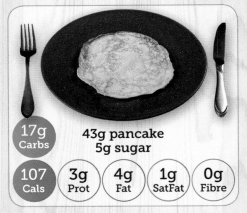

17g Carbs

43g pancake
5g sugar

107 Cals **3g** Prot **4g** Fat **1g** SatFat **0g** Fibre

Breakfast Tart

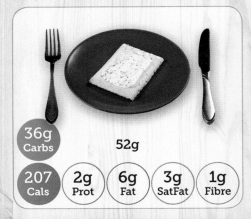

36g Carbs

52g

207 Cals **2g** Prot **6g** Fat **3g** SatFat **1g** Fibre

Scotch Pancake

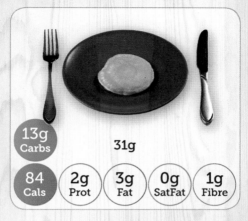

13g Carbs

31g

84 Cals | 2g Prot | 3g Fat | 0g SatFat | 1g Fibre

Eggy Bread

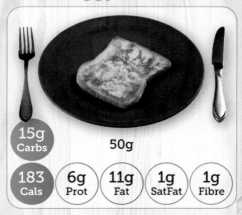

15g Carbs

50g

183 Cals | 6g Prot | 11g Fat | 1g SatFat | 1g Fibre

Fried Bread (in oil)

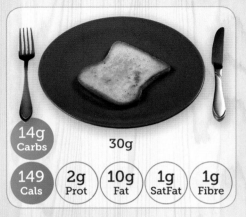

14g Carbs

30g

149 Cals | **2g** Prot | **10g** Fat | **1g** SatFat | **1g** Fibre

Waffle (sweet)

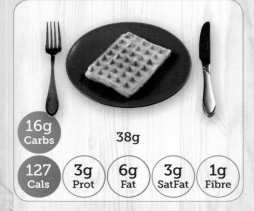

16g Carbs

38g

127 Cals | **3g** Prot | **6g** Fat | **3g** SatFat | **1g** Fibre

Bakewell Tart

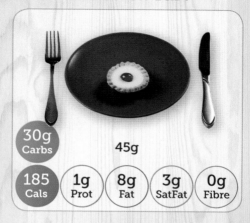

30g Carbs

45g

185 Cals   **1g** Prot   **8g** Fat   **3g** SatFat   **0g** Fibre

Baklava

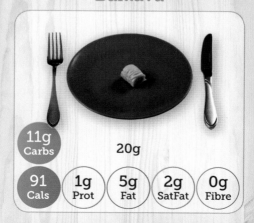

11g Carbs

20g

91 Cals   **1g** Prot   **5g** Fat   **2g** SatFat   **0g** Fibre

Carrot Cake

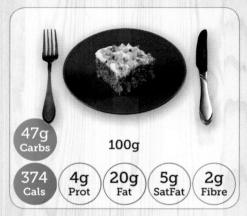

47g Carbs

100g

374 Cals | **4g** Prot | **20g** Fat | **5g** SatFat | **2g** Fibre

Chocolate Cake

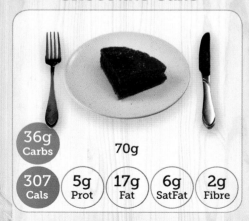

36g Carbs

70g

307 Cals | **5g** Prot | **17g** Fat | **6g** SatFat | **2g** Fibre

Coffee & Walnut Cake

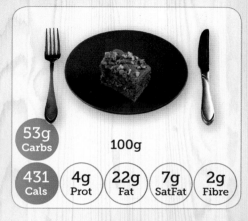

53g Carbs

100g

431 Cals | **4g** Prot | **22g** Fat | **7g** SatFat | **2g** Fibre

Fruit Cake

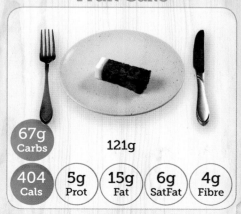

67g Carbs

121g

404 Cals | **5g** Prot | **15g** Fat | **6g** SatFat | **4g** Fibre

Ginger Cake

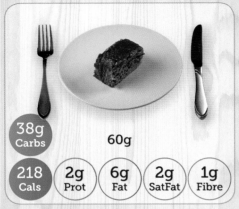

38g Carbs

60g

218 Cals

2g Prot

6g Fat

2g SatFat

1g Fibre

Malt Loaf

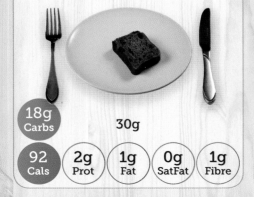

18g Carbs

30g

92 Cals

2g Prot

1g Fat

0g SatFat

1g Fibre

Swiss Roll

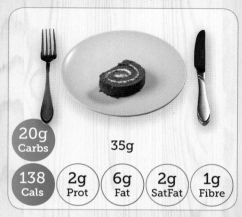

20g
Carbs

35g

138
Cals

2g
Prot

6g
Fat

2g
SatFat

1g
Fibre

Victoria Sponge

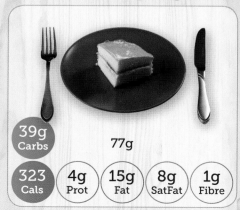

39g
Carbs

77g

323
Cals

4g
Prot

15g
Fat

8g
SatFat

1g
Fibre

Apple Danish

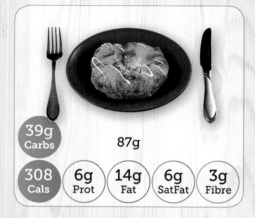

39g Carbs

87g

308 Cals

6g Prot

14g Fat

6g SatFat

3g Fibre

Chocolate Chip Twist

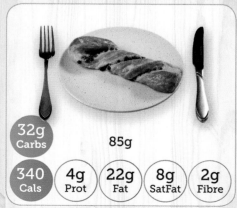

32g Carbs

85g

340 Cals

4g Prot

22g Fat

8g SatFat

2g Fibre

Cinnamon Swirl

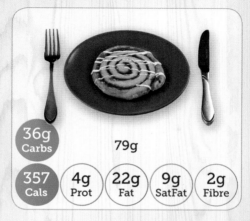

36g Carbs

79g

357 Cals | **4g** Prot | **22g** Fat | **9g** SatFat | **2g** Fibre

Fruit Trellis

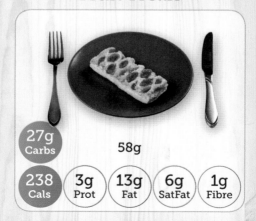

27g Carbs

58g

238 Cals | **3g** Prot | **13g** Fat | **6g** SatFat | **1g** Fibre

Pain aux Raisins

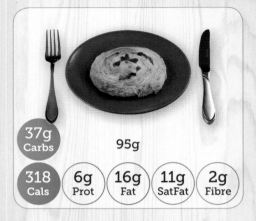

37g Carbs

95g

318 Cals

6g Prot

16g Fat

11g SatFat

2g Fibre

Pecan Plait

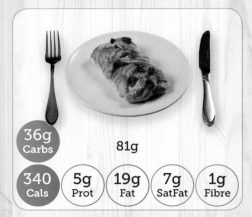

36g Carbs

81g

340 Cals

5g Prot

19g Fat

7g SatFat

1g Fibre

Chocolate Éclair

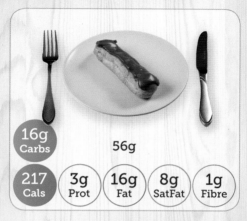

16g Carbs

56g

217 Cals

3g Prot

16g Fat

8g SatFat

1g Fibre

Corn Flake Cake

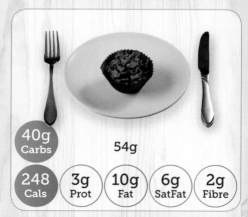

40g Carbs

54g

248 Cals

3g Prot

10g Fat

6g SatFat

2g Fibre

Cup Cake

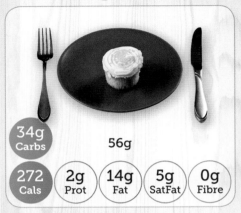

34g Carbs

272 Cals

56g

2g Prot

14g Fat

5g SatFat

0g Fibre

Custard Slice

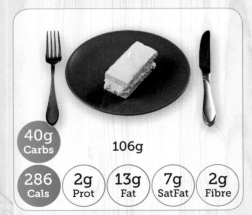

40g Carbs

286 Cals

106g

2g Prot

13g Fat

7g SatFat

2g Fibre

Custard Tart

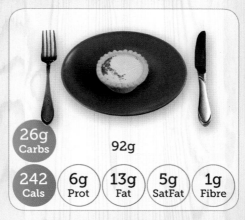

26g Carbs

92g

242 Cals

6g Prot

13g Fat

5g SatFat

1g Fibre

Mini Battenburg

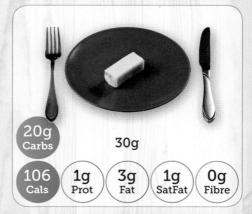

20g Carbs

30g

106 Cals

1g Prot

3g Fat

1g SatFat

0g Fibre

Choc Ring Doughnut

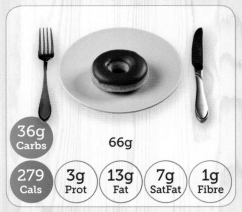

36g Carbs

66g

279 Cals

3g Prot

13g Fat

7g SatFat

1g Fibre

Glazed Ring Doughnut

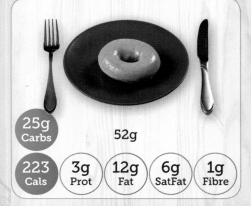

25g Carbs

52g

223 Cals

3g Prot

12g Fat

6g SatFat

1g Fibre

Jam Doughnut

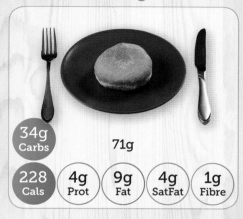

34g Carbs

71g

228 Cals | **4g** Prot | **9g** Fat | **4g** SatFat | **1g** Fibre

Mini Doughnut

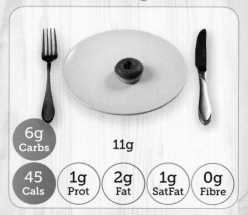

6g Carbs

11g

45 Cals | **1g** Prot | **2g** Fat | **1g** SatFat | **0g** Fibre

Sprinkle Ring Doughnut

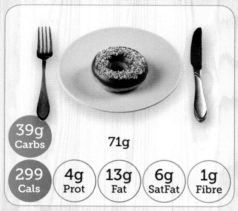

39g Carbs

71g

299 Cals | **4g** Prot | **13g** Fat | **6g** SatFat | **1g** Fibre

Sugar Ring Doughnut

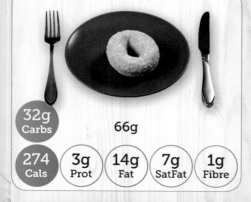

32g Carbs

66g

274 Cals | **3g** Prot | **14g** Fat | **7g** SatFat | **1g** Fibre

Fresh Cream Doughnut

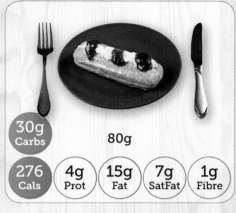

30g Carbs

80g

276 Cals | **4g** Prot | **15g** Fat | **7g** SatFat | **1g** Fibre

Yum Yum

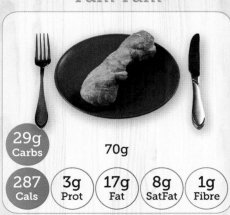

29g Carbs

70g

287 Cals | **3g** Prot | **17g** Fat | **8g** SatFat | **1g** Fibre

Blueberry Muffin

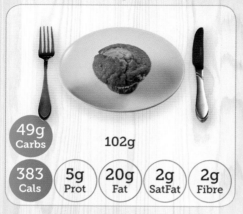

49g Carbs

102g

383 Cals

5g Prot

20g Fat

2g SatFat

2g Fibre

Chocolate Muffin

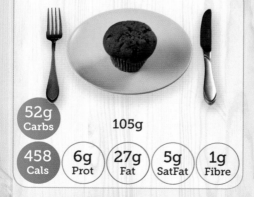

52g Carbs

105g

458 Cals

6g Prot

27g Fat

5g SatFat

1g Fibre

Flapjack

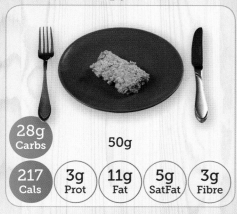

28g Carbs

50g

217 Cals

3g Prot

11g Fat

5g SatFat

3g Fibre

Meringue Nest

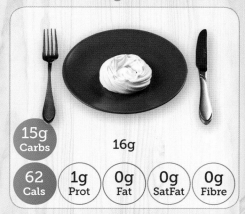

15g Carbs

16g

62 Cals

1g Prot

0g Fat

0g SatFat

0g Fibre

Mince Pie

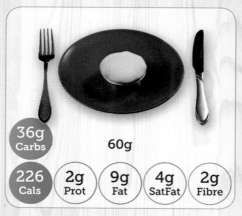

36g Carbs

60g

226 Cals

2g Prot

9g Fat

4g SatFat

2g Fibre

Belgian Bun

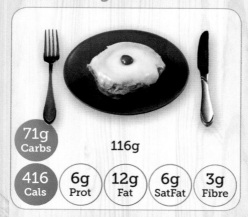

71g Carbs

116g

416 Cals

6g Prot

12g Fat

6g SatFat

3g Fibre

Iced Bun

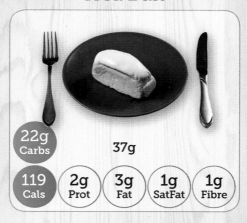

22g Carbs

37g

119 Cals   2g Prot   3g Fat   1g SatFat   1g Fibre

Hot Cross Bun

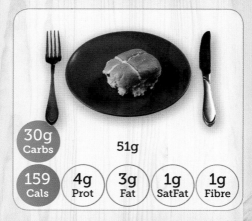

30g Carbs

51g

159 Cals   4g Prot   3g Fat   1g SatFat   1g Fibre

Cheese Scone

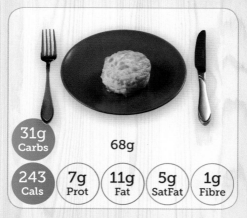

31g Carbs

68g

243 Cals

7g Prot

11g Fat

5g SatFat

1g Fibre

Fruit Scone

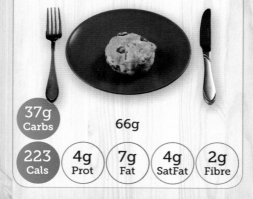

37g Carbs

66g

223 Cals

4g Prot

7g Fat

4g SatFat

2g Fibre

Brie

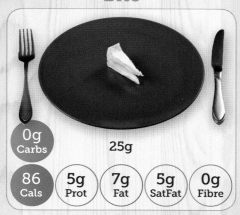

0g
Carbs

25g

86
Cals

5g
Prot

7g
Fat

5g
SatFat

0g
Fibre

Camembert

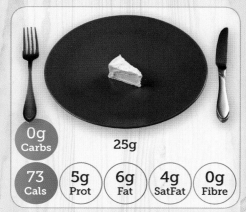

0g
Carbs

25g

73
Cals

5g
Prot

6g
Fat

4g
SatFat

0g
Fibre

Cheddar

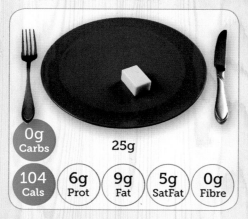

0g Carbs

25g

104 Cals | 6g Prot | 9g Fat | 5g SatFat | 0g Fibre

Cheddar (reduced fat)

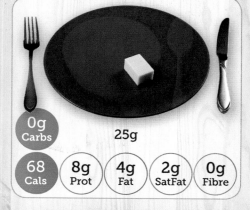

0g Carbs

25g

68 Cals | 8g Prot | 4g Fat | 2g SatFat | 0g Fibre

Cheddar (grated)

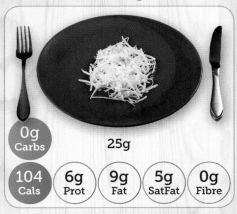

0g Carbs

25g

104 Cals | 6g Prot | 9g Fat | 5g SatFat | 0g Fibre

Cheddar (sliced)

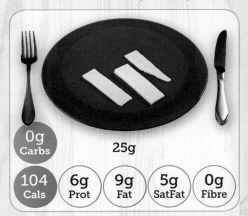

0g Carbs

25g

104 Cals | 6g Prot | 9g Fat | 5g SatFat | 0g Fibre

Cottage Cheese

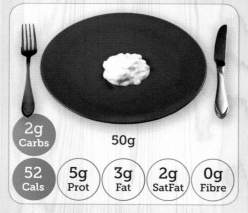

2g
Carbs

50g

52
Cals

5g
Prot

3g
Fat

2g
SatFat

0g
Fibre

Cream Cheese

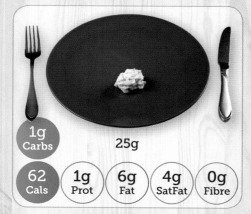

1g
Carbs

25g

62
Cals

1g
Prot

6g
Fat

4g
SatFat

0g
Fibre

Edam

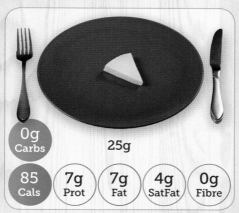

25g

0g
Carbs

85
Cals

7g
Prot

7g
Fat

4g
SatFat

0g
Fibre

Feta

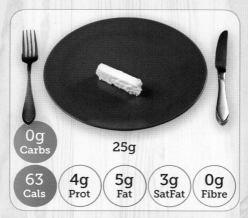

25g

0g
Carbs

63
Cals

4g
Prot

5g
Fat

3g
SatFat

0g
Fibre

Goat's Cheese

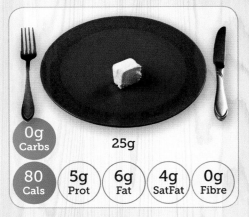

0g
Carbs

25g

80
Cals

5g
Prot

6g
Fat

4g
SatFat

0g
Fibre

Halloumi

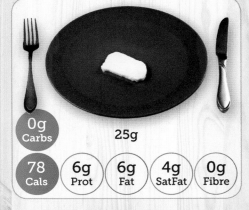

0g
Carbs

25g

78
Cals

6g
Prot

6g
Fat

4g
SatFat

0g
Fibre

Mozzarella

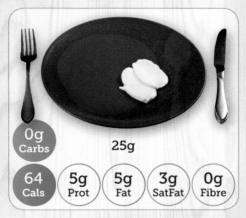

0g Carbs

25g

64 Cals

5g Prot

5g Fat

3g SatFat

0g Fibre

Parmesan

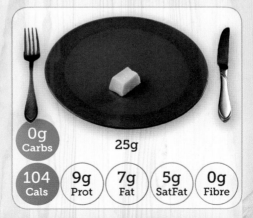

0g Carbs

25g

104 Cals

9g Prot

7g Fat

5g SatFat

0g Fibre

Parmesan (grated)

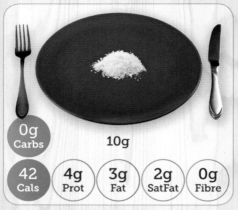

0g Carbs

10g

42 Cals | 4g Prot | 3g Fat | 2g SatFat | 0g Fibre

Ricotta

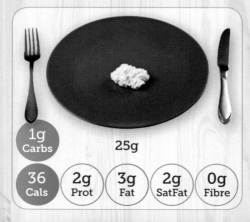

1g Carbs

25g

36 Cals | 2g Prot | 3g Fat | 2g SatFat | 0g Fibre

Squirty Cheese

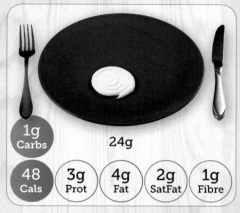

1g Carbs

24g

48 Cals | 3g Prot | 4g Fat | 2g SatFat | 1g Fibre

Spreadable Cheese

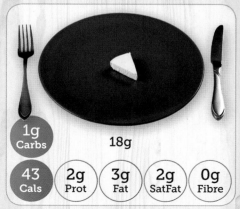

1g Carbs

18g

43 Cals | 2g Prot | 3g Fat | 2g SatFat | 0g Fibre

Processed Cheese Slice

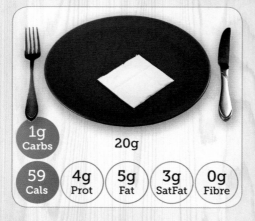

1g Carbs

20g

59 Cals | 4g Prot | 5g Fat | 3g SatFat | 0g Fibre

Stilton

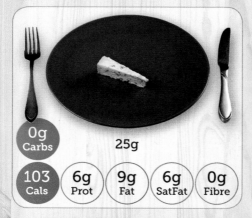

0g Carbs

25g

103 Cals | 6g Prot | 9g Fat | 6g SatFat | 0g Fibre

Red Leicester

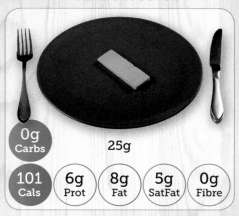

0g
Carbs

25g

101
Cals

6g
Prot

8g
Fat

5g
SatFat

0g
Fibre

Wensleydale with Cranberries

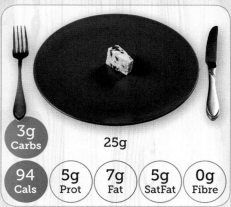

3g
Carbs

25g

94
Cals

5g
Prot

7g
Fat

5g
SatFat

0g
Fibre

Apple Pie

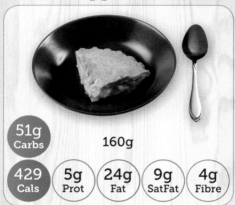

51g Carbs

160g

429 Cals · **5g** Prot · **24g** Fat · **9g** SatFat · **4g** Fibre

Apple & Rhubarb Crumble

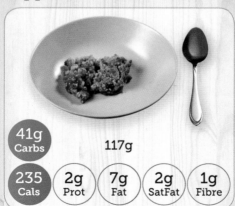

41g Carbs

117g

235 Cals · **2g** Prot · **7g** Fat · **2g** SatFat · **1g** Fibre

Apple Strudel

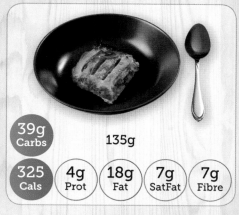

39g Carbs

135g

325 Cals

4g Prot

18g Fat

7g SatFat

7g Fibre

Banoffee Pie

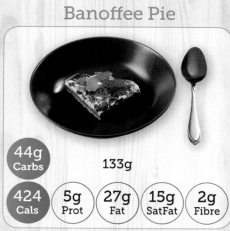

44g Carbs

133g

424 Cals

5g Prot

27g Fat

15g SatFat

2g Fibre

Black Forest Gateau

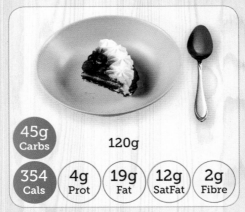

45g Carbs

120g

354 Cals

4g Prot

19g Fat

12g SatFat

2g Fibre

Bread & Butter Pudding

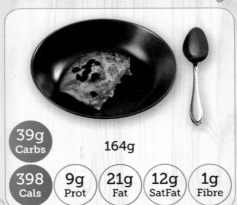

39g Carbs

164g

398 Cals

9g Prot

21g Fat

12g SatFat

1g Fibre

Brownie

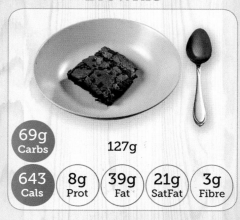

69g Carbs

127g

643 Cals | **8g** Prot | **39g** Fat | **21g** SatFat | **3g** Fibre

Cheesecake

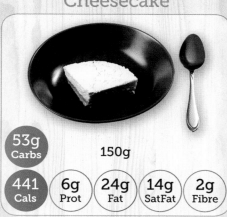

53g Carbs

150g

441 Cals | **6g** Prot | **24g** Fat | **14g** SatFat | **2g** Fibre

Chocolate Mousse

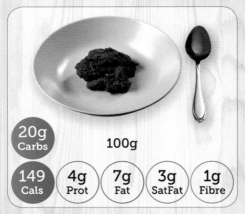

20g Carbs

100g

149 Cals

4g Prot

7g Fat

3g SatFat

1g Fibre

Chocolate Torte

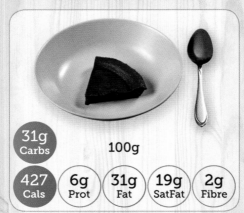

31g Carbs

100g

427 Cals

6g Prot

31g Fat

19g SatFat

2g Fibre

Christmas Pudding

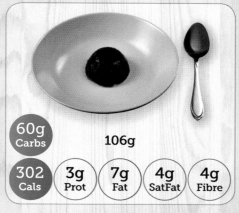

60g Carbs

106g

302 Cals | **3g** Prot | **7g** Fat | **4g** SatFat | **4g** Fibre

Custard
(with semi-skimmed milk)

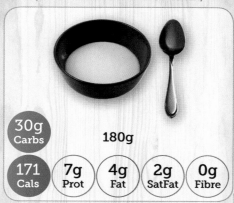

30g Carbs

180g

171 Cals | **7g** Prot | **4g** Fat | **2g** SatFat | **0g** Fibre

Ice Cream (chocolate)

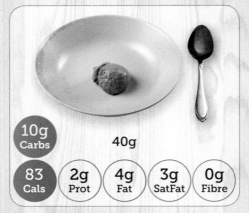

10g Carbs

40g

83 Cals | **2g** Prot | **4g** Fat | **3g** SatFat | **0g** Fibre

Ice Cream (vanilla)

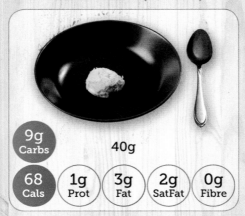

9g Carbs

40g

68 Cals | **1g** Prot | **3g** Fat | **2g** SatFat | **0g** Fibre

Sorbet (lemon)

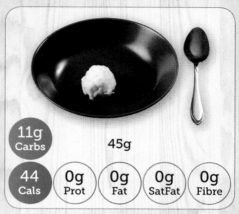

11g Carbs

45g

44 Cals | **0g** Prot | **0g** Fat | **0g** SatFat | **0g** Fibre

Sorbet (raspberry)

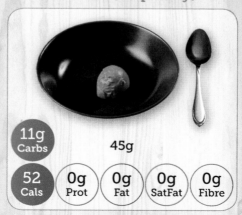

11g Carbs

45g

52 Cals | **0g** Prot | **0g** Fat | **0g** SatFat | **0g** Fibre

Choc Ice

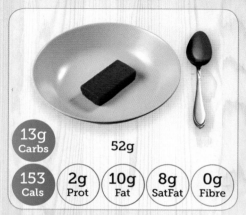

13g Carbs

52g

153 Cals

2g Prot

10g Fat

8g SatFat

0g Fibre

Crème Brûlée

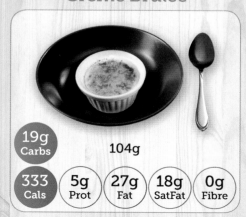

19g Carbs

104g

333 Cals

5g Prot

27g Fat

18g SatFat

0g Fibre

Chocolate & Nut Cone

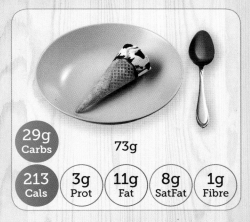

29g Carbs

73g

213 Cals

3g Prot

11g Fat

8g SatFat

1g Fibre

Panna Cotta

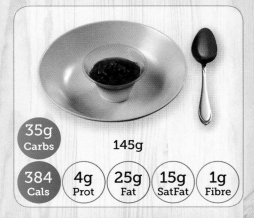

35g Carbs

145g

384 Cals

4g Prot

25g Fat

15g SatFat

1g Fibre

Ice Cream Lolly

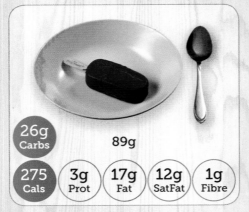

26g Carbs

89g

275 Cals   **3g** Prot   **17g** Fat   **12g** SatFat   **1g** Fibre

Strawberry Tartlet

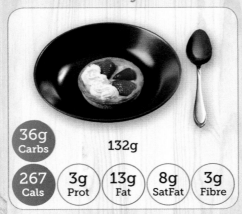

36g Carbs

132g

267 Cals   **3g** Prot   **13g** Fat   **8g** SatFat   **3g** Fibre

Jelly

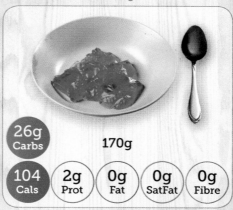

26g Carbs

170g

104 Cals | **2g** Prot | **0g** Fat | **0g** SatFat | **0g** Fibre

Jelly (sugar free)

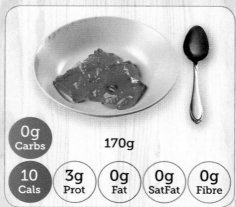

0g Carbs

170g

10 Cals | **3g** Prot | **0g** Fat | **0g** SatFat | **0g** Fibre

Lemon Meringue Pie

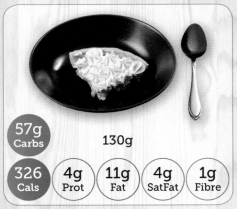

57g Carbs

130g

326 Cals

4g Prot

11g Fat

4g SatFat

1g Fibre

Profiteroles

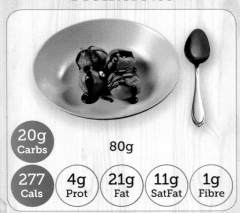

20g Carbs

80g

277 Cals

4g Prot

21g Fat

11g SatFat

1g Fibre

Rice Pudding

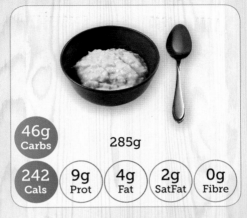

46g Carbs

285g

242 Cals

9g Prot

4g Fat

2g SatFat

0g Fibre

Roulade

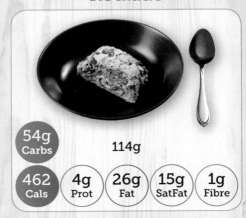

54g Carbs

114g

462 Cals

4g Prot

26g Fat

15g SatFat

1g Fibre

Spotted Dick

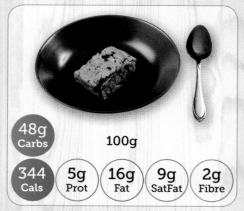

48g Carbs

100g

344 Cals

5g Prot

16g Fat

9g SatFat

2g Fibre

Sticky Toffee Pudding

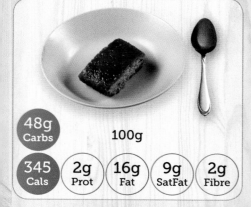

48g Carbs

100g

345 Cals

2g Prot

16g Fat

9g SatFat

2g Fibre

Strawberry Delight

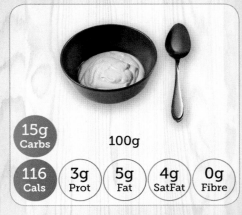

15g Carbs

100g

116 Cals | **3g** Prot | **5g** Fat | **4g** SatFat | **0g** Fibre

Summer Pudding

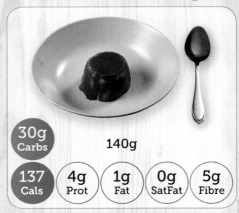

30g Carbs

140g

137 Cals | **4g** Prot | **1g** Fat | **0g** SatFat | **5g** Fibre

Tiramisu

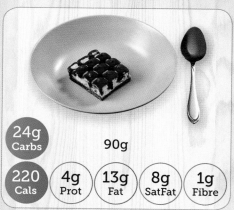

24g Carbs

90g

220 Cals

4g Prot

13g Fat

8g SatFat

1g Fibre

Trifle

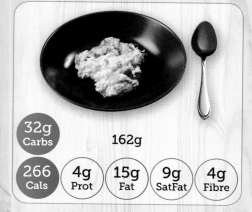

32g Carbs

162g

266 Cals

4g Prot

15g Fat

9g SatFat

4g Fibre

Apple Juice

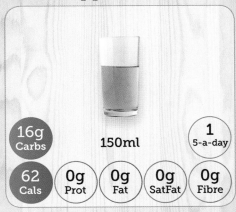

16g Carbs

150ml

1 5-a-day

62 Cals

0g Prot

0g Fat

0g SatFat

0g Fibre

Cranberry Juice

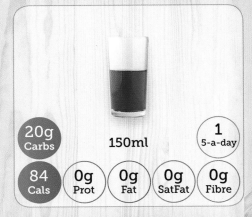

20g Carbs

150ml

1 5-a-day

84 Cals

0g Prot

0g Fat

0g SatFat

0g Fibre

Grapefruit Juice

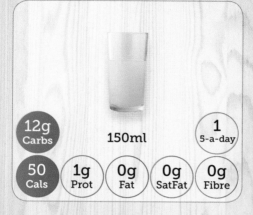

12g
Carbs

150ml

1
5-a-day

50
Cals

1g
Prot

0g
Fat

0g
SatFat

0g
Fibre

Orange Juice

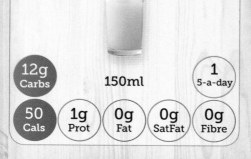

12g
Carbs

150ml

1
5-a-day

50
Cals

1g
Prot

0g
Fat

0g
SatFat

0g
Fibre

Pineapple Juice

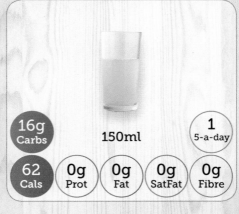

16g Carbs

150ml

1 5-a-day

62 Cals | **0g** Prot | **0g** Fat | **0g** SatFat | **0g** Fibre

Tomato Juice

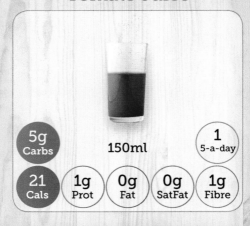

5g Carbs

150ml

1 5-a-day

21 Cals | **1g** Prot | **0g** Fat | **0g** SatFat | **1g** Fibre

Squash

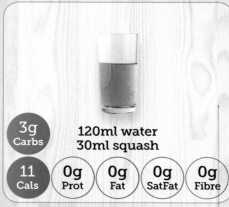

3g Carbs

120ml water
30ml squash

11 Cals

0g Prot

0g Fat

0g SatFat

0g Fibre

Squash
(no added sugar)

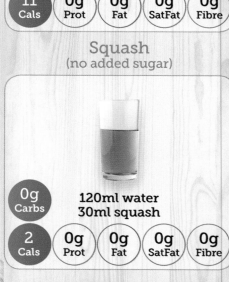

0g Carbs

120ml water
30ml squash

2 Cals

0g Prot

0g Fat

0g SatFat

0g Fibre

Cola

31g Carbs

284ml, half pint

116 Cals

0g Prot

0g Fat

0g SatFat

0g Fibre

Diet Cola

0g Carbs

284ml, half pint

3 Cals

0g Prot

0g Fat

0g SatFat

0g Fibre

Lemonade (sparkling)

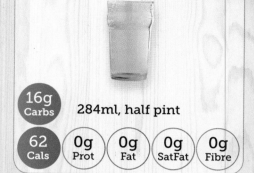

16g Carbs

284ml, half pint

62 Cals

0g Prot

0g Fat

0g SatFat

0g Fibre

Lemonade (fresh)

47g Carbs

284ml, half pint

179 Cals

0g Prot

0g Fat

0g SatFat

0g Fibre

Lucozade Energy

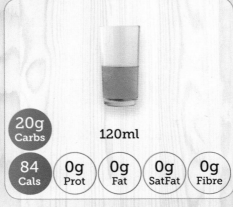

20g Carbs

120ml

84 Cals | **0g** Prot | **0g** Fat | **0g** SatFat | **0g** Fibre

Iced Tea

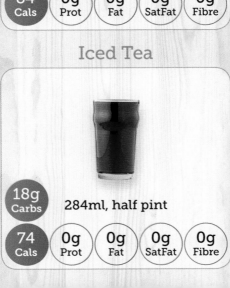

18g Carbs

284ml, half pint

74 Cals | **0g** Prot | **0g** Fat | **0g** SatFat | **0g** Fibre

Malt Drink

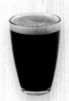

50g Carbs

330ml, bottle

201 Cals | **0g** Prot | **0g** Fat | **0g** SatFat | **0g** Fibre

Smoothie
(strawberry & banana)

18g Carbs

150ml

1½ 5-a-day

74 Cals | **1g** Prot | **0g** Fat | **0g** SatFat | **2g** Fibre

Cappuccino
(whole milk)

10g
Carbs

355ml, 12 fl oz

116
Cals

6g
Prot

6g
Fat

3g
SatFat

0g
Fibre

Cappuccino
(skimmed milk)

11g
Carbs

355ml, 12 fl oz

70
Cals

7g
Prot

0g
Fat

0g
SatFat

0g
Fibre

Hot Chocolate
(whole milk)

38g Carbs

355ml, 12 fl oz

316 Cals | **13g** Prot | **13g** Fat | **9g** SatFat | **0g** Fibre

Hot Chocolate
(skimmed milk)

39g Carbs

355ml, 12 fl oz

220 Cals | **13g** Prot | **2g** Fat | **1g** SatFat | **0g** Fibre

Latte
(whole milk)

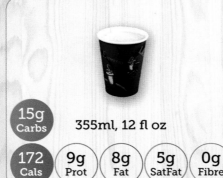

15g Carbs

355ml, 12 fl oz

172 Cals | **9g** Prot | **8g** Fat | **5g** SatFat | **0g** Fibre

Latte
(skimmed milk)

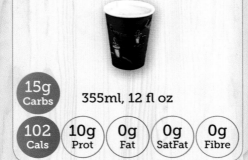

15g Carbs

355ml, 12 fl oz

102 Cals | **10g** Prot | **0g** Fat | **0g** SatFat | **0g** Fibre

Cup of Coffee (black)

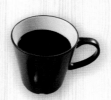

1g Carbs

260ml

5 Cals | **1g** Prot | **0g** Fat | **0g** SatFat | **0g** Fibre

Cup of Coffee (with milk)

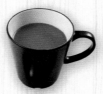

2g Carbs

260ml

18 Cals | **2g** Prot | **1g** Fat | **0g** SatFat | **0g** Fibre

Cup of Tea (with milk)

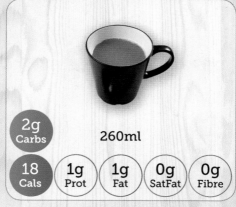

2g Carbs

260ml

18 Cals | **1g** Prot | **1g** Fat | **0g** SatFat | **0g** Fibre

Espresso

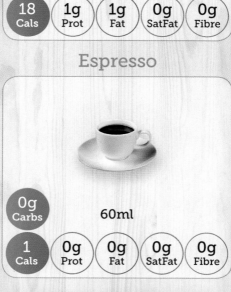

0g Carbs

60ml

1 Cals | **0g** Prot | **0g** Fat | **0g** SatFat | **0g** Fibre

Hot Malt Drink

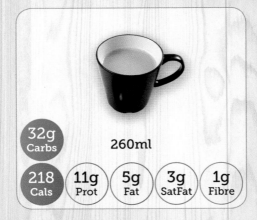

32g Carbs

260ml

218 Cals | **11g** Prot | **5g** Fat | **3g** SatFat | **1g** Fibre

Teaspoon of Sugar

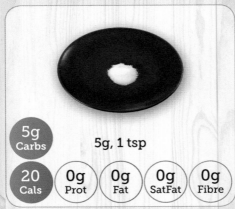

5g Carbs

5g, 1 tsp

20 Cals | **0g** Prot | **0g** Fat | **0g** SatFat | **0g** Fibre

Ale (4% ABV)

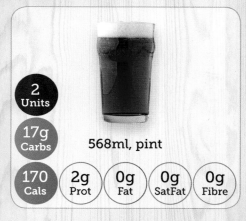

2 Units

17g Carbs

568ml, pint

170 Cals

2g Prot

0g Fat

0g SatFat

0g Fibre

Lager (4% ABV)

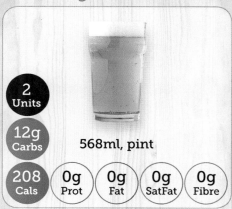

2 Units

12g Carbs

568ml, pint

208 Cals

0g Prot

0g Fat

0g SatFat

0g Fibre

Stout (4% ABV)

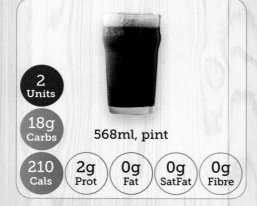

2 Units

18g Carbs

568ml, pint

210 Cals

2g Prot

0g Fat

0g SatFat

0g Fibre

Cider (dry, 5% ABV)

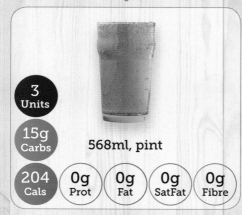

3 Units

15g Carbs

568ml, pint

204 Cals

0g Prot

0g Fat

0g SatFat

0g Fibre

Cider (sweet, 5% ABV)

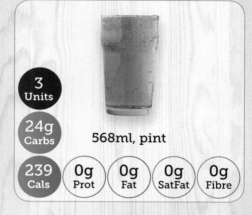

3 Units

24g Carbs

239 Cals

568ml, pint

0g Prot	0g Fat	0g SatFat	0g Fibre

WKD Vodka Blue

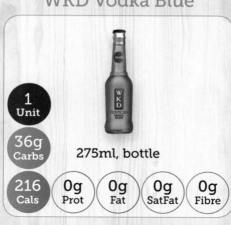

1 Unit

36g Carbs

216 Cals

275ml, bottle

0g Prot	0g Fat	0g SatFat	0g Fibre

WKD Iron Brew

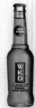

1 Unit

22g Carbs

275ml, bottle

161 Cals

0g Prot

0g Fat

0g SatFat

0g Fibre

Red Wine

3 Units

1g Carbs

250ml, large glass

190 Cals

0g Prot

0g Fat

0g SatFat

0g Fibre

White Wine (dry)

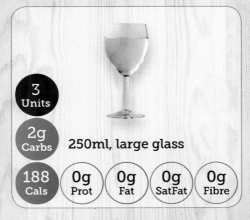

3 Units

2g Carbs 250ml, large glass

188 Cals | **0g Prot** | **0g Fat** | **0g SatFat** | **0g Fibre**

Sweet White Wine

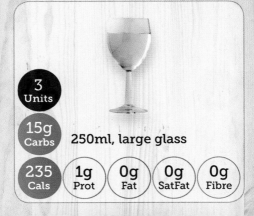

3 Units

15g Carbs 250ml, large glass

235 Cals | **1g Prot** | **0g Fat** | **0g SatFat** | **0g Fibre**

Champagne

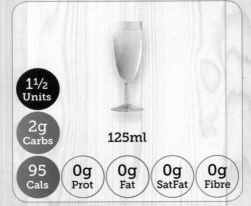

1½ Units

2g Carbs

95 Cals

125ml

0g Prot **0g Fat** **0g SatFat** **0g Fibre**

Advocaat

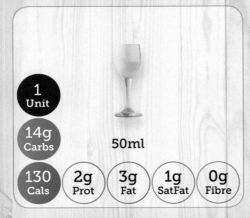

1 Unit

14g Carbs

130 Cals

50ml

2g Prot **3g Fat** **1g SatFat** **0g Fibre**

Irish Cream

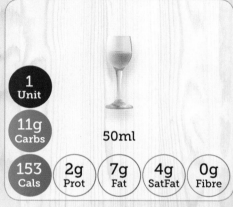

1 Unit

11g Carbs

153 Cals

50ml

2g Prot

7g Fat

4g SatFat

0g Fibre

Port

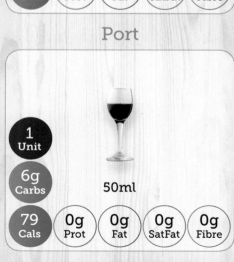

1 Unit

6g Carbs

79 Cals

50ml

0g Prot

0g Fat

0g SatFat

0g Fibre

Sherry

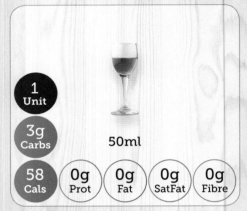

1 Unit

3g Carbs

50ml

58 Cals

0g Prot

0g Fat

0g SatFat

0g Fibre

Vermouth (sweet)

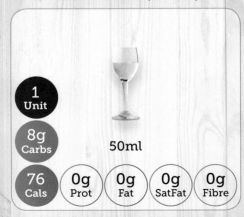

1 Unit

8g Carbs

50ml

76 Cals

0g Prot

0g Fat

0g SatFat

0g Fibre

Brandy

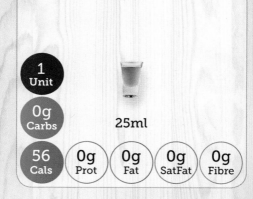

1 Unit

0g Carbs

56 Cals

0g Prot

0g Fat

0g SatFat

0g Fibre

25ml

Gin

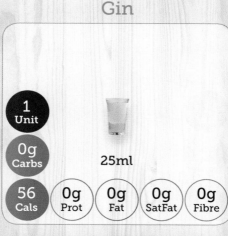

1 Unit

0g Carbs

56 Cals

0g Prot

0g Fat

0g SatFat

0g Fibre

25ml

Rum

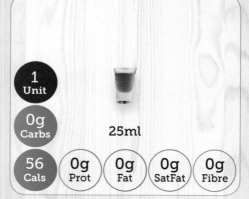

1
Unit

0g
Carbs

56
Cals

25ml

0g
Prot

0g
Fat

0g
SatFat

0g
Fibre

Sweet Liqueur

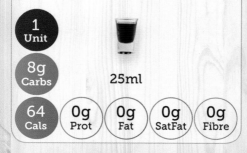

1
Unit

8g
Carbs

64
Cals

25ml

0g
Prot

0g
Fat

0g
SatFat

0g
Fibre

Vodka

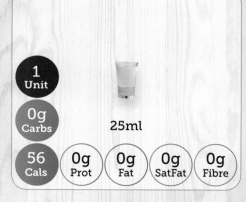

1 Unit

0g Carbs

56 Cals

25ml

0g Prot

0g Fat

0g SatFat

0g Fibre

Whisky

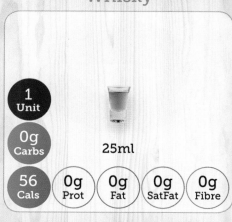

1 Unit

0g Carbs

56 Cals

25ml

0g Prot

0g Fat

0g SatFat

0g Fibre

Boiled Egg

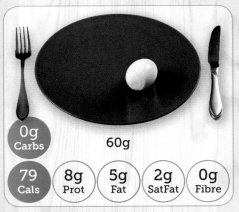

0g Carbs

60g

79 Cals | 8g Prot | 5g Fat | 2g SatFat | 0g Fibre

Fried Egg

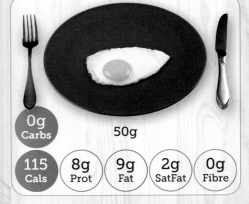

0g Carbs

50g

115 Cals | 8g Prot | 9g Fat | 2g SatFat | 0g Fibre

Poached Egg

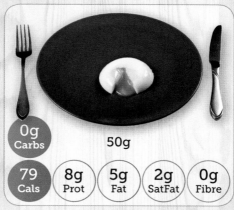

0g
Carbs

50g

79
Cals

8g
Prot

5g
Fat

2g
SatFat

0g
Fibre

Scotch Egg

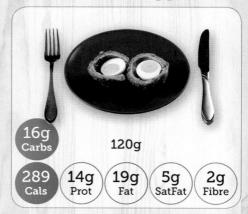

16g
Carbs

120g

289
Cals

14g
Prot

19g
Fat

5g
SatFat

2g
Fibre

Scrambled Egg (with milk)

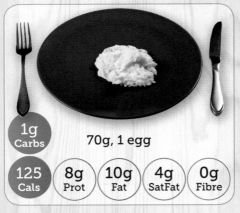

1g Carbs

70g, 1 egg

125 Cals

8g Prot

10g Fat

4g SatFat

0g Fibre

Scrambled Egg (with milk)

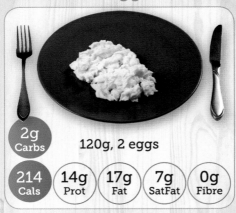

2g Carbs

120g, 2 eggs

214 Cals

14g Prot

17g Fat

7g SatFat

0g Fibre

Omelette (plain)

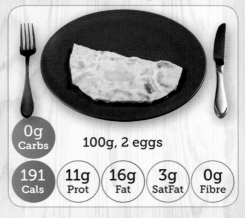

0g Carbs

100g, 2 eggs

191 Cals | 11g Prot | 16g Fat | 3g SatFat | 0g Fibre

Omelette (cheese)

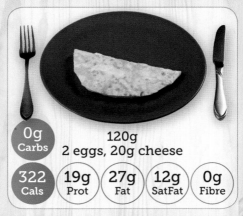

0g Carbs

120g
2 eggs, 20g cheese

322 Cals | 19g Prot | 27g Fat | 12g SatFat | 0g Fibre

Eggs Benedict

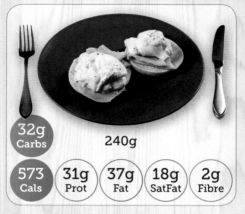

32g Carbs

240g

573 Cals

31g Prot

37g Fat

18g SatFat

2g Fibre

Eggs Florentine

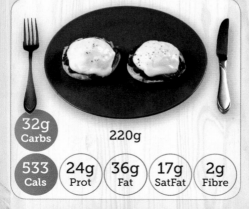

32g Carbs

220g

533 Cals

24g Prot

36g Fat

17g SatFat

2g Fibre

Apricots

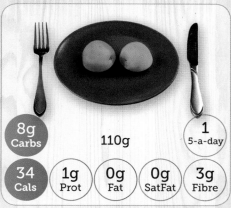

8g Carbs

110g

1 5-a-day

34 Cals

1g Prot

0g Fat

0g SatFat

3g Fibre

Apricots (tinned in juice)

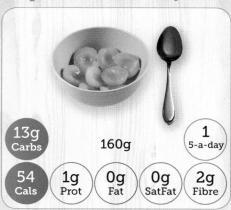

13g Carbs

160g

1 5-a-day

54 Cals

1g Prot

0g Fat

0g SatFat

2g Fibre

Apple

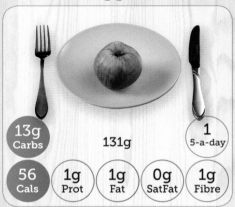

13g Carbs

131g

1 5-a-day

56 Cals

1g Prot

1g Fat

0g SatFat

1g Fibre

Blackberries

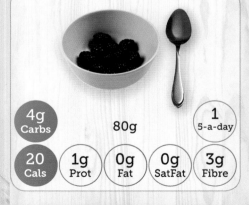

4g Carbs

80g

1 5-a-day

20 Cals

1g Prot

0g Fat

0g SatFat

3g Fibre

Banana (with skin)

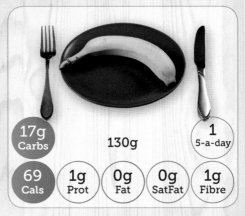

17g Carbs

130g

1 5-a-day

69 Cals

1g Prot

0g Fat

0g SatFat

1g Fibre

Banana (without skin)

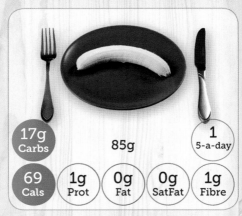

17g Carbs

85g

1 5-a-day

69 Cals

1g Prot

0g Fat

0g SatFat

1g Fibre

Blueberries

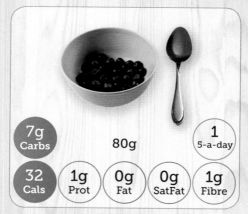

7g Carbs

80g

1 5-a-day

32 Cals

1g Prot

0g Fat

0g SatFat

1g Fibre

Cherries

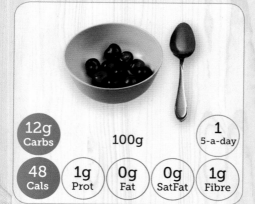

12g Carbs

100g

1 5-a-day

48 Cals

1g Prot

0g Fat

0g SatFat

1g Fibre

Clementine

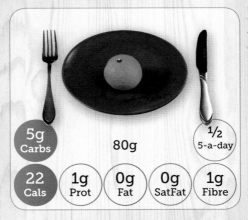

5g Carbs

80g

1/2 5-a-day

22 Cals

1g Prot

0g Fat

0g SatFat

1g Fibre

Cranberries

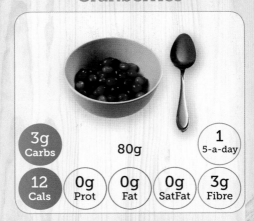

3g Carbs

80g

1 5-a-day

12 Cals

0g Prot

0g Fat

0g SatFat

3g Fibre

Figs

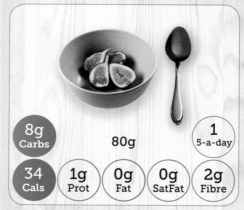

8g Carbs

80g

1 5-a-day

34 Cals

1g Prot

0g Fat

0g SatFat

2g Fibre

Fruit Cocktail
(tinned in juice)

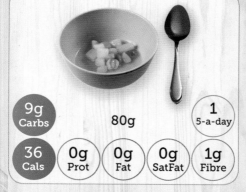

9g Carbs

80g

1 5-a-day

36 Cals

0g Prot

0g Fat

0g SatFat

1g Fibre

Grapefruit

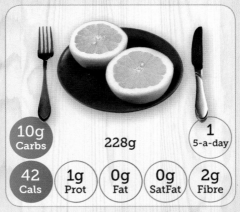

10g Carbs

228g

1 5-a-day

42 Cals

1g Prot

0g Fat

0g SatFat

2g Fibre

Grapes (seedless)

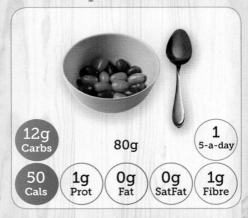

12g Carbs

80g

1 5-a-day

50 Cals

1g Prot

0g Fat

0g SatFat

1g Fibre

Kiwi

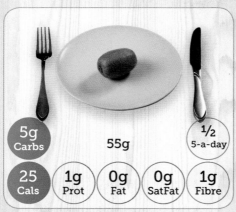

5g Carbs

55g

1/2 5-a-day

25 Cals

1g Prot

0g Fat

0g SatFat

1g Fibre

Mango

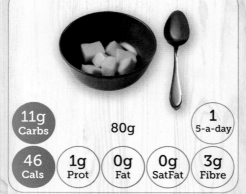

11g Carbs

80g

1 5-a-day

46 Cals

1g Prot

0g Fat

0g SatFat

3g Fibre

Melon (honeydew)

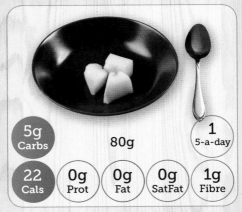

5g Carbs

80g

1 5-a-day

22 Cals

0g Prot

0g Fat

0g SatFat

1g Fibre

Orange

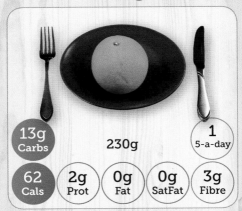

13g Carbs

230g

1 5-a-day

62 Cals

2g Prot

0g Fat

0g SatFat

3g Fibre

Papaya

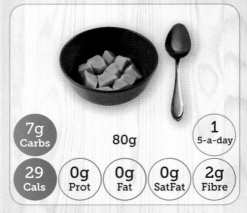

7g Carbs

80g

1 5-a-day

29 Cals

0g Prot

0g Fat

0g SatFat

2g Fibre

Pomegranate

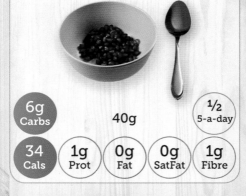

6g Carbs

40g

½ 5-a-day

34 Cals

1g Prot

0g Fat

0g SatFat

1g Fibre

Peach

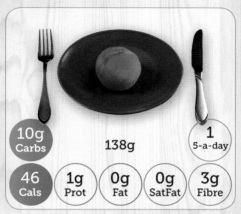

10g Carbs

138g

1 5-a-day

46 Cals | 1g Prot | 0g Fat | 0g SatFat | 3g Fibre

Peaches (tinned in juice)

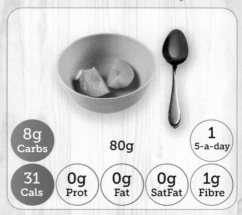

8g Carbs

80g

1 5-a-day

31 Cals | 0g Prot | 0g Fat | 0g SatFat | 1g Fibre

Nectarine

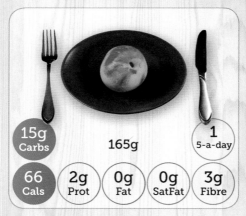

15g Carbs

165g

1 5-a-day

66 Cals

2g Prot

0g Fat

0g SatFat

3g Fibre

Pear

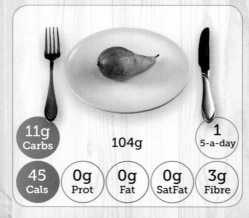

11g Carbs

104g

1 5-a-day

45 Cals

0g Prot

0g Fat

0g SatFat

3g Fibre

Pears (tinned in juice)

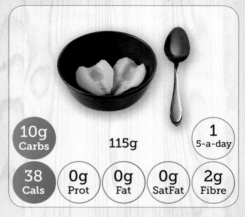

10g Carbs

115g

1 5-a-day

38 Cals | 0g Prot | 0g Fat | 0g SatFat | 2g Fibre

Persimmon

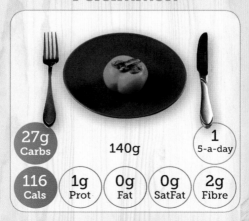

27g Carbs

140g

1 5-a-day

116 Cals | 1g Prot | 0g Fat | 0g SatFat | 2g Fibre

Pineapple

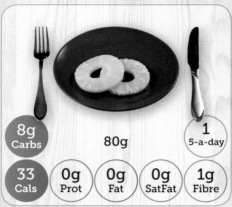

8g Carbs

80g

1 5-a-day

33 Cals

0g Prot

0g Fat

0g SatFat

1g Fibre

Pineapple (tinned in juice)

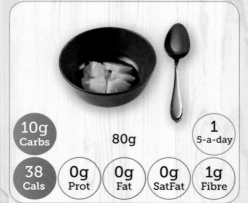

10g Carbs

80g

1 5-a-day

38 Cals

0g Prot

0g Fat

0g SatFat

1g Fibre

Plum

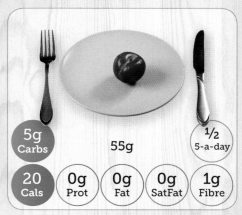

5g Carbs

55g

1/2 5-a-day

20 Cals

0g Prot

0g Fat

0g SatFat

1g Fibre

Raspberries

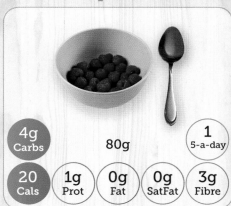

4g Carbs

80g

1 5-a-day

20 Cals

1g Prot

0g Fat

0g SatFat

3g Fibre

Rhubarb (stewed with sugar)

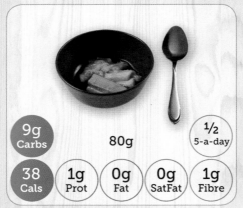

9g Carbs

80g

½ 5-a-day

38 Cals

1g Prot

0g Fat

0g SatFat

1g Fibre

Satsuma

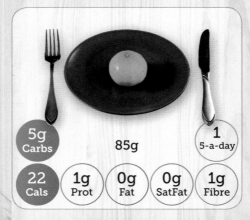

5g Carbs

85g

1 5-a-day

22 Cals

1g Prot

0g Fat

0g SatFat

1g Fibre

Strawberries

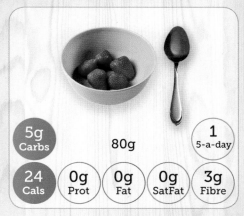

5g
Carbs

80g

1
5-a-day

24
Cals

0g
Prot

0g
Fat

0g
SatFat

3g
Fibre

Watermelon

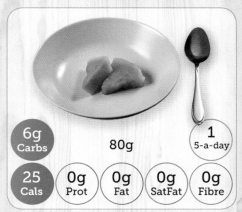

6g
Carbs

80g

1
5-a-day

25
Cals

0g
Prot

0g
Fat

0g
SatFat

0g
Fibre

Apple Rings

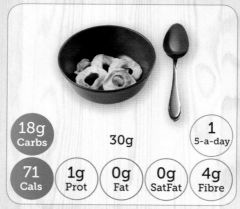

18g Carbs

30g

1 5-a-day

71 Cals

1g Prot

0g Fat

0g SatFat

4g Fibre

Apricots

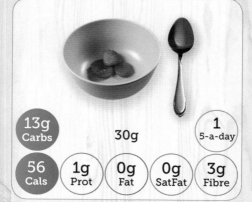

13g Carbs

30g

1 5-a-day

56 Cals

1g Prot

0g Fat

0g SatFat

3g Fibre

Banana Chips

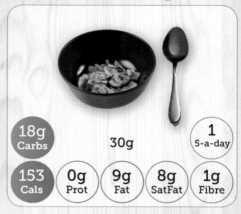

18g Carbs

30g

1 5-a-day

153 Cals

0g Prot

9g Fat

8g SatFat

1g Fibre

Cranberries

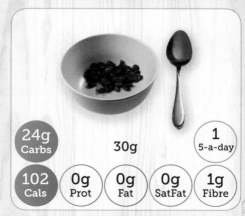

24g Carbs

30g

1 5-a-day

102 Cals

0g Prot

0g Fat

0g SatFat

1g Fibre

Dates

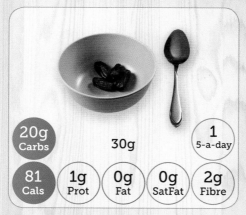

20g Carbs

30g

1 5-a-day

81 Cals

1g Prot

0g Fat

0g SatFat

2g Fibre

Figs

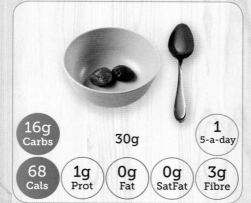

16g Carbs

30g

1 5-a-day

68 Cals

1g Prot

0g Fat

0g SatFat

3g Fibre

Pineapple

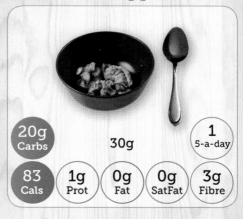

20g Carbs

30g

1 5-a-day

83 Cals

1g Prot

0g Fat

0g SatFat

3g Fibre

Prunes

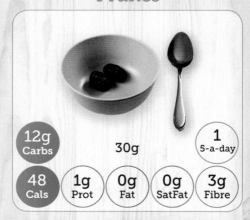

12g Carbs

30g

1 5-a-day

48 Cals

1g Prot

0g Fat

0g SatFat

3g Fibre

Raisins

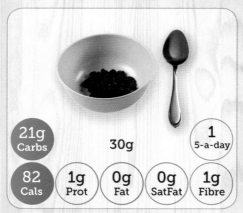

21g Carbs

30g

1 5-a-day

82 Cals

1g Prot

0g Fat

0g SatFat

1g Fibre

Sultanas

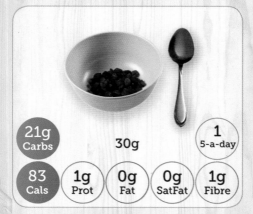

21g Carbs

30g

1 5-a-day

83 Cals

1g Prot

0g Fat

0g SatFat

1g Fibre

Fibre Flakes GF

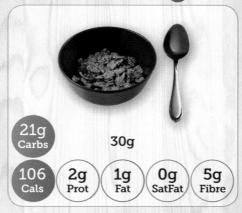

21g Carbs

30g

106 Cals | **2g** Prot | **1g** Fat | **0g** SatFat | **5g** Fibre

Special Flakes GF

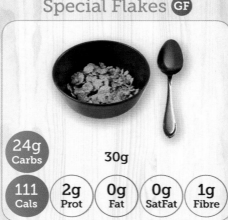

24g Carbs

30g

111 Cals | **2g** Prot | **0g** Fat | **0g** SatFat | **1g** Fibre

Muesli GF

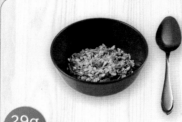

29g Carbs

50g

186 Cals

5g Prot

5g Fat

1g SatFat

4g Fibre

Porridge GF
(with skimmed milk)

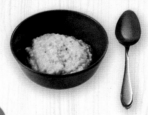

33g Carbs

220g (27g oats)

246 Cals

13g Prot

7g Fat

3g SatFat

3g Fibre

Brown Bread GF
(home baked)

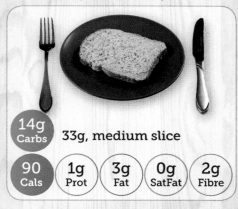

14g Carbs

33g, medium slice

90 Cals | **1g** Prot | **3g** Fat | **0g** SatFat | **2g** Fibre

White Bread GF
(home baked)

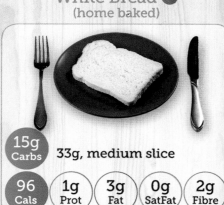

15g Carbs

33g, medium slice

96 Cals | **1g** Prot | **3g** Fat | **0g** SatFat | **2g** Fibre

Brown Bread (sliced) GF

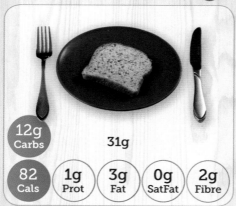

12g Carbs

31g

82 Cals | 1g Prot | 3g Fat | 0g SatFat | 2g Fibre

White Bread (sliced) GF

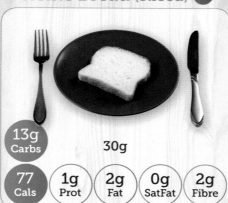

13g Carbs

30g

77 Cals | 1g Prot | 2g Fat | 0g SatFat | 2g Fibre

Fibre Roll **GF**

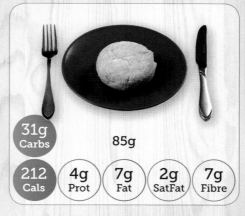

31g Carbs

85g

212 Cals | **4g** Prot | **7g** Fat | **2g** SatFat | **7g** Fibre

White Roll **GF**

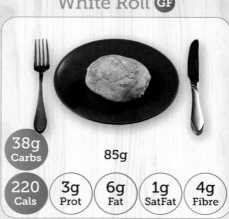

38g Carbs

85g

220 Cals | **3g** Prot | **6g** Fat | **1g** SatFat | **4g** Fibre

Brown Roll (part baked) GF

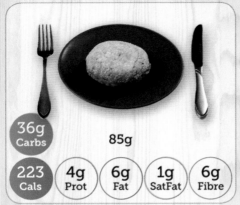

36g Carbs

85g

223 Cals | **4g** Prot | **6g** Fat | **1g** SatFat | **6g** Fibre

White Roll (part baked) GF

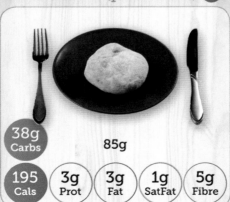

38g Carbs

85g

195 Cals | **3g** Prot | **3g** Fat | **1g** SatFat | **5g** Fibre

Breadstick GF

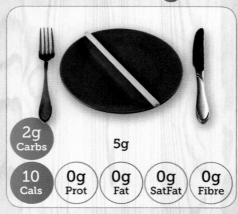

2g Carbs

5g

10 Cals | 0g Prot | 0g Fat | 0g SatFat | 0g Fibre

Crispbread GF

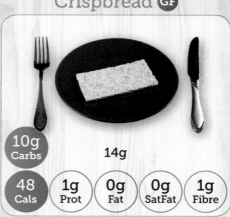

10g Carbs

14g

48 Cals | 1g Prot | 0g Fat | 0g SatFat | 1g Fibre

Naan Bread GF

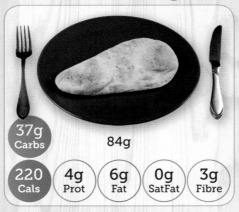

37g Carbs

84g

220 Cals | **4g** Prot | **6g** Fat | **0g** SatFat | **3g** Fibre

Pitta Bread GF

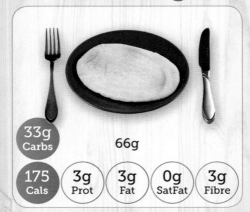

33g Carbs

66g

175 Cals | **3g** Prot | **3g** Fat | **0g** SatFat | **3g** Fibre

Pizza Base GF

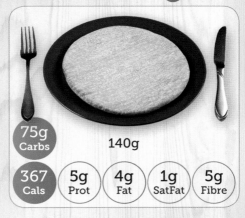

75g Carbs

140g

367 Cals | **5g** Prot | **4g** Fat | **1g** SatFat | **5g** Fibre

Rice Cake GF

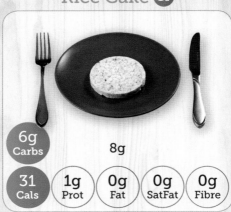

6g Carbs

8g

31 Cals | **1g** Prot | **0g** Fat | **0g** SatFat | **0g** Fibre

Chocolate Chip Cookie GF

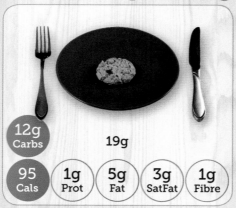

12g Carbs

19g

95 Cals

1g Prot

5g Fat

3g SatFat

1g Fibre

Chocolate Digestive GF

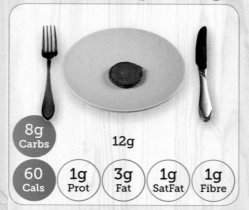

8g Carbs

12g

60 Cals

1g Prot

3g Fat

1g SatFat

1g Fibre

Digestive GF

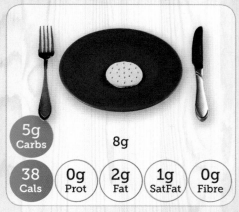

5g Carbs

8g

38 Cals | 0g Prot | 2g Fat | 1g SatFat | 0g Fibre

Savoury Biscuit GF

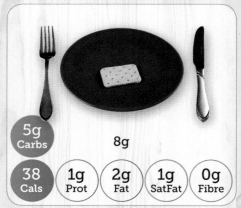

5g Carbs

8g

38 Cals | 1g Prot | 2g Fat | 1g SatFat | 0g Fibre

Sweet Biscuit GF

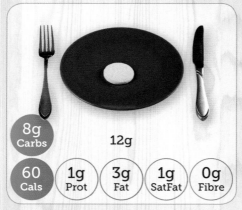

8g Carbs

12g

60 Cals | 1g Prot | 3g Fat | 1g SatFat | 0g Fibre

Tea Biscuit GF

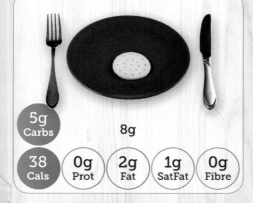

5g Carbs

8g

38 Cals | 0g Prot | 2g Fat | 1g SatFat | 0g Fibre

Pasta Twists GF

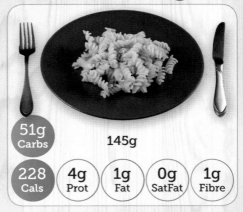

51g
Carbs

145g

228
Cals

4g
Prot

1g
Fat

0g
SatFat

1g
Fibre

Penne (fibre) GF

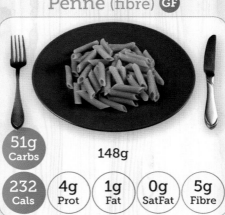

51g
Carbs

148g

232
Cals

4g
Prot

1g
Fat

0g
SatFat

5g
Fibre

Spaghetti GF

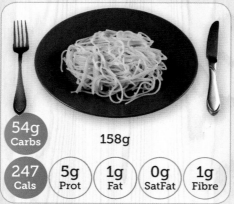

54g Carbs

158g

247 Cals

5g Prot

1g Fat

0g SatFat

1g Fibre

Tagliatelle GF

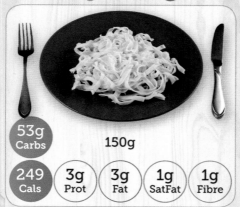

53g Carbs

150g

249 Cals

3g Prot

3g Fat

1g SatFat

1g Fibre

Beans on Toast (with butter)

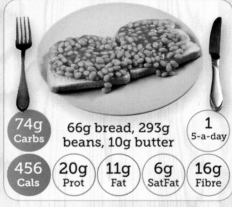

74g Carbs

66g bread, 293g beans, 10g butter

1 5-a-day

456 Cals | **20g** Prot | **11g** Fat | **6g** SatFat | **16g** Fibre

Chicken Goujons, Potato Smiles & Peas

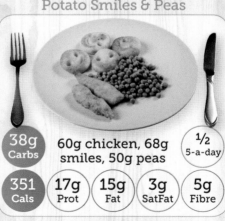

38g Carbs

60g chicken, 68g smiles, 50g peas

½ 5-a-day

351 Cals | **17g** Prot | **15g** Fat | **3g** SatFat | **5g** Fibre

Fish Fingers, Chips & Baked Beans

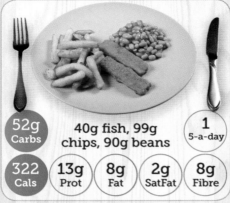

52g Carbs

40g fish, 99g chips, 90g beans

1 5-a-day

322 Cals | **13g** Prot | **8g** Fat | **2g** SatFat | **8g** Fibre

Beef Stew & Dumplings

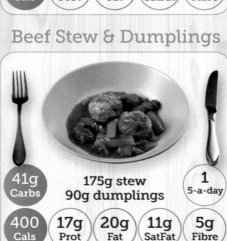

41g Carbs

175g stew 90g dumplings

1 5-a-day

400 Cals | **17g** Prot | **20g** Fat | **11g** SatFat | **5g** Fibre

Corned Beef Hash

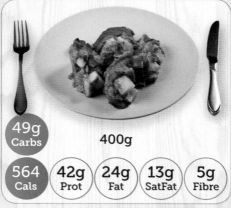

49g Carbs

400g

564 Cals

42g Prot

24g Fat

13g SatFat

5g Fibre

Chilli con Carne
(with White Rice)

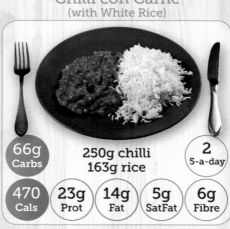

66g Carbs

250g chilli
163g rice

2 5-a-day

470 Cals

23g Prot

14g Fat

5g SatFat

6g Fibre

Curry, Chicken
(with White Rice)

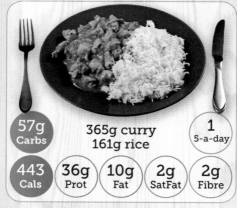

57g Carbs

365g curry
161g rice

1 5-a-day

443 Cals | **36g** Prot | **10g** Fat | **2g** SatFat | **2g** Fibre

Curry, Lentil
(with Brown Rice)

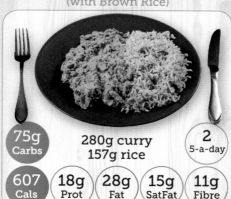

75g Carbs

280g curry
157g rice

2 5-a-day

607 Cals | **18g** Prot | **28g** Fat | **15g** SatFat | **11g** Fibre

Curry, Vegetable & Potato
(with White Rice)

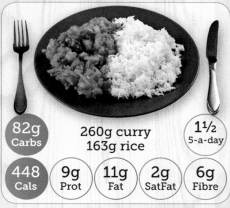

82g Carbs

260g curry
163g rice

1½ 5-a-day

448 Cals

9g Prot

11g Fat

2g SatFat

6g Fibre

Fish Pie

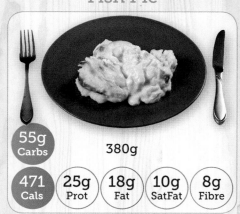

55g Carbs

380g

471 Cals

25g Prot

18g Fat

10g SatFat

8g Fibre

Fish Stew with Jollof Rice

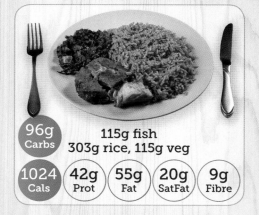

96g Carbs

115g fish
303g rice, 115g veg

1024 Cals | **42g** Prot | **55g** Fat | **20g** SatFat | **9g** Fibre

Caribbean Dumplings

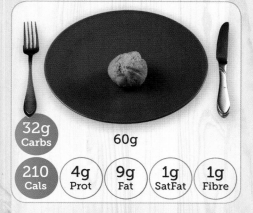

32g Carbs

60g

210 Cals | **4g** Prot | **9g** Fat | **1g** SatFat | **1g** Fibre

Jamaican Beef Patty

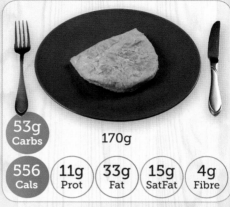

53g Carbs

170g

556 Cals | **11g** Prot | **33g** Fat | **15g** SatFat | **4g** Fibre

Goat & Potato Curry
(with Rice & Peas)

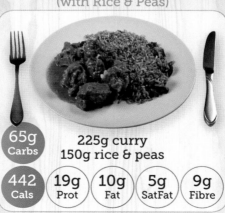

65g Carbs

225g curry
150g rice & peas

442 Cals | **19g** Prot | **10g** Fat | **5g** SatFat | **9g** Fibre

Jerk Chicken
(with Rice & Peas)

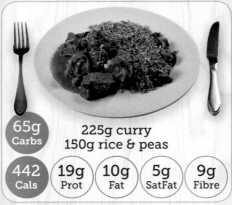

65g Carbs

225g curry
150g rice & peas

442 Cals

19g Prot

10g Fat

5g SatFat

9g Fibre

Fried Fish (with Rice & Peas)

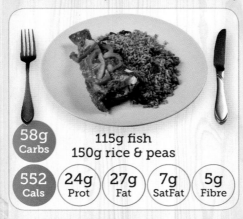

58g Carbs

115g fish
150g rice & peas

552 Cals

24g Prot

27g Fat

7g SatFat

5g Fibre

Lasagne

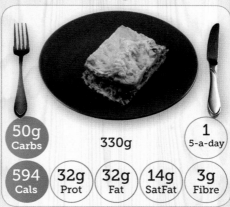

50g Carbs

330g

1 5-a-day

594 Cals

32g Prot

32g Fat

14g SatFat

3g Fibre

Veggie Lasagne

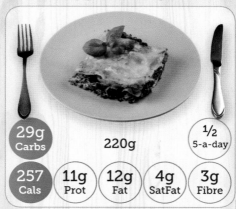

29g Carbs

220g

½ 5-a-day

257 Cals

11g Prot

12g Fat

4g SatFat

3g Fibre

Mushroom Risotto

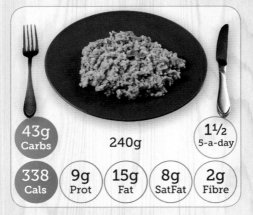

43g Carbs

240g

1½ 5-a-day

338 Cals

9g Prot

15g Fat

8g SatFat

2g Fibre

Macaroni Cheese

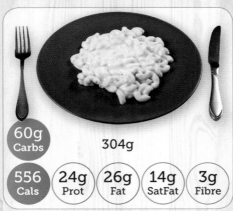

60g Carbs

304g

556 Cals

24g Prot

26g Fat

14g SatFat

3g Fibre

Penne Arrabbiata

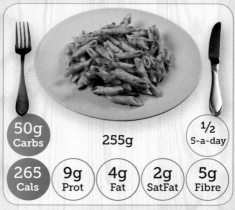

50g
Carbs

255g

1/2
5-a-day

265
Cals

9g
Prot

4g
Fat

2g
SatFat

5g
Fibre

Pasta Bake
(tuna, sweetcorn & cheese)

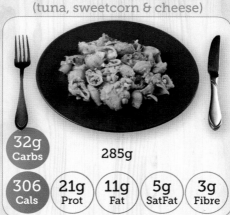

32g
Carbs

285g

306
Cals

21g
Prot

11g
Fat

5g
SatFat

3g
Fibre

Pasta Meal
(chicken, broccoli & mascarpone)

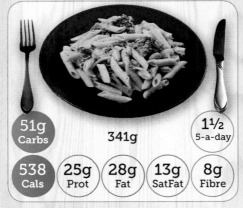

51g Carbs

341g

1½ 5-a-day

538 Cals

25g Prot

28g Fat

13g SatFat

8g Fibre

Chicken & Bacon Pie

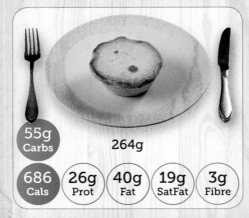

55g Carbs

264g

686 Cals

26g Prot

40g Fat

19g SatFat

3g Fibre

Steak Pie

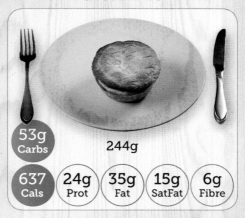

53g Carbs

244g

637 Cals

24g Prot

35g Fat

15g SatFat

6g Fibre

Steak & Potato Pie

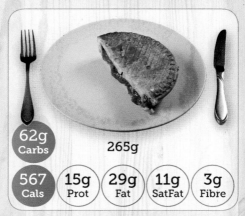

62g Carbs

265g

567 Cals

15g Prot

29g Fat

11g SatFat

3g Fibre

Steak & Kidney Pudding

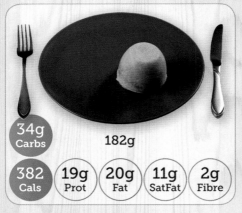

34g Carbs

182g

382 Cals

19g Prot

20g Fat

11g SatFat

2g Fibre

Top Crust Pie

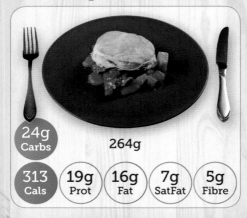

24g Carbs

264g

313 Cals

19g Prot

16g Fat

7g SatFat

5g Fibre

Pizza
(chicken, deep pan, oven baked)

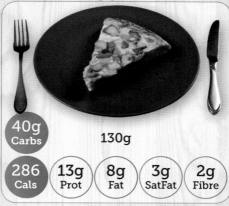

40g Carbs

130g

286 Cals

13g Prot

8g Fat

3g SatFat

2g Fibre

Pizza
(pepperoni, thin crust, oven baked)

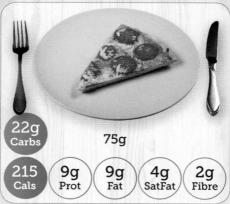

22g Carbs

75g

215 Cals

9g Prot

9g Fat

4g SatFat

2g Fibre

Quiche Lorraine

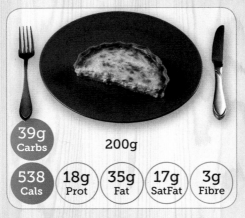

39g Carbs

200g

538 Cals

18g Prot

35g Fat

17g SatFat

3g Fibre

Salmon Frittata

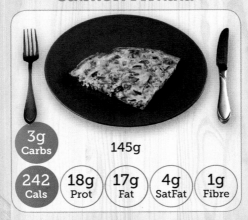

3g Carbs

145g

242 Cals

18g Prot

17g Fat

4g SatFat

1g Fibre

Chicken Caesar Salad

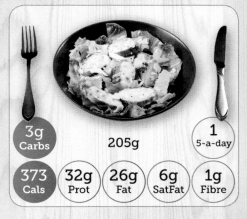

3g Carbs

205g

1 5-a-day

373 Cals

32g Prot

26g Fat

6g SatFat

1g Fibre

Greek Salad

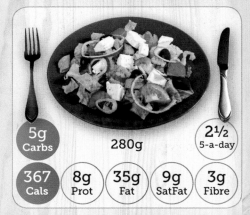

5g Carbs

280g

2½ 5-a-day

367 Cals

8g Prot

35g Fat

9g SatFat

3g Fibre

Tuna Niçoise Salad

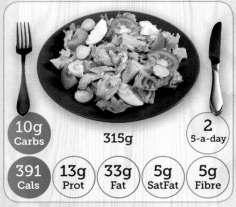

10g Carbs

315g

2 5-a-day

391 Cals

13g Prot

33g Fat

5g SatFat

5g Fibre

Sausage & Mash
(with butter)

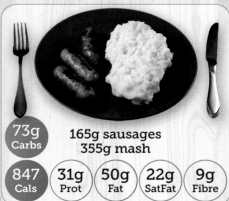

73g Carbs

165g sausages
355g mash

847 Cals

31g Prot

50g Fat

22g SatFat

9g Fibre

Shepherd's Pie

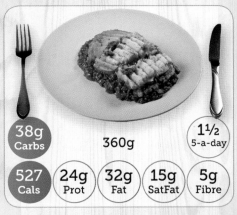

38g Carbs

360g

1½ 5-a-day

527 Cals

24g Prot

32g Fat

15g SatFat

5g Fibre

Spaghetti Bolognese

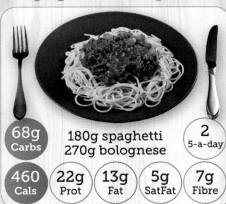

68g Carbs

180g spaghetti
270g bolognese

2 5-a-day

460 Cals

22g Prot

13g Fat

5g SatFat

7g Fibre

Spaghetti Carbonara

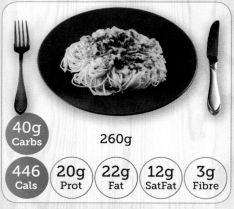

40g Carbs

260g

446 Cals | **20g** Prot | **22g** Fat | **12g** SatFat | **3g** Fibre

Stir Fry
(cashew, without noodles)

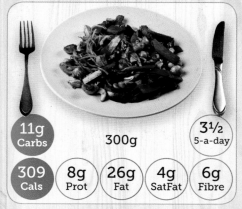

11g Carbs

300g

3½ 5-a-day

309 Cals | **8g** Prot | **26g** Fat | **4g** SatFat | **6g** Fibre

Stir Fry
(chicken & noodles)

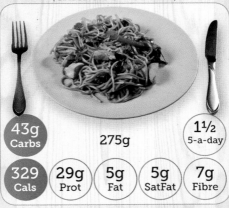

43g Carbs

275g

1½ 5-a-day

329 Cals

29g Prot

5g Fat

5g SatFat

7g Fibre

Toad in the Hole

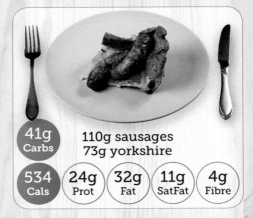

41g Carbs

110g sausages
73g yorkshire

534 Cals

24g Prot

32g Fat

11g SatFat

4g Fibre

Coleslaw

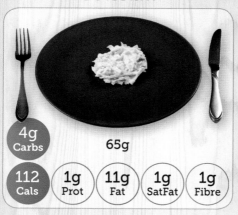

4g Carbs

65g

112 Cals

1g Prot

11g Fat

1g SatFat

1g Fibre

Gherkins

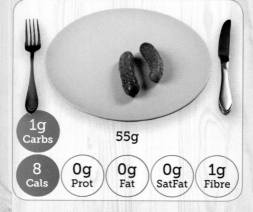

1g Carbs

55g

8 Cals

0g Prot

0g Fat

0g SatFat

1g Fibre

Olives (pitted in brine)

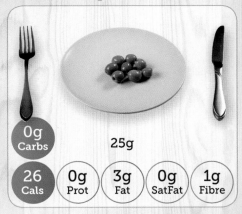

0g
Carbs

25g

26
Cals

0g
Prot

3g
Fat

0g
SatFat

1g
Fibre

Onion Rings (battered)

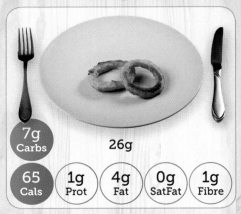

7g
Carbs

26g

65
Cals

1g
Prot

4g
Fat

0g
SatFat

1g
Fibre

Pickled Onions

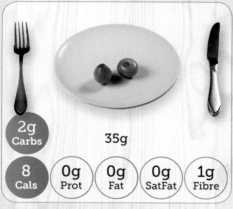

2g Carbs

35g

8 Cals

0g Prot

0g Fat

0g SatFat

1g Fibre

Sun-dried Tomatoes
(in oil, drained)

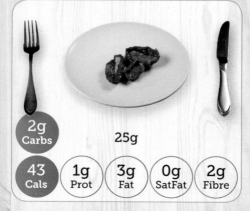

2g Carbs

25g

43 Cals

1g Prot

3g Fat

0g SatFat

2g Fibre

Stuffing (packet mix)

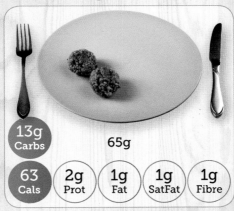

13g Carbs

65g

63 Cals

2g Prot

1g Fat

1g SatFat

1g Fibre

Yorkshire Pudding

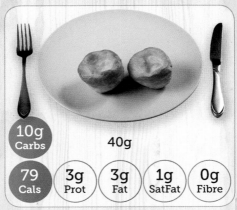

10g Carbs

40g

79 Cals

3g Prot

3g Fat

1g SatFat

0g Fibre

Cornish Pasty

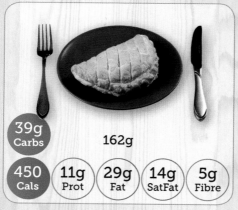

39g Carbs

162g

450 Cals

11g Prot

29g Fat

14g SatFat

5g Fibre

Pork Pie

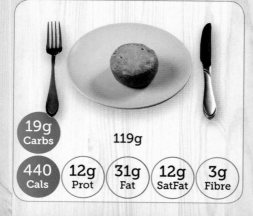

19g Carbs

119g

440 Cals

12g Prot

31g Fat

12g SatFat

3g Fibre

Sausage Roll

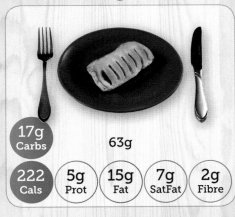

17g Carbs

63g

222 Cals

5g Prot

15g Fat

7g SatFat

2g Fibre

Sausages & Beans (tinned)

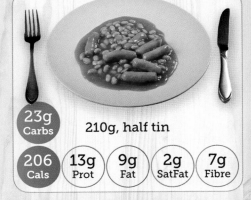

23g Carbs

210g, half tin

206 Cals

13g Prot

9g Fat

2g SatFat

7g Fibre

Haggis

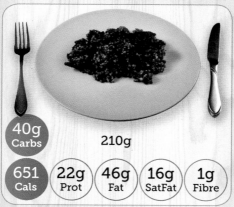

40g Carbs

210g

651 Cals

22g Prot

46g Fat

16g SatFat

1g Fibre

Black Pudding (dry fried)

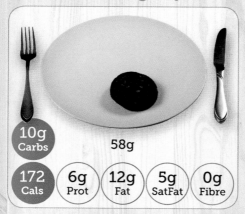

10g Carbs

58g

172 Cals

6g Prot

12g Fat

5g SatFat

0g Fibre

Chicken Goujon (baked)

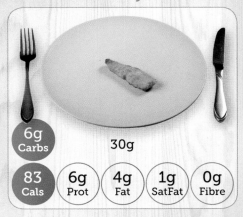

6g
Carbs

30g

83
Cals

6g
Prot

4g
Fat

1g
SatFat

0g
Fibre

Brussels Pâté

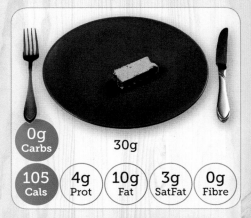

0g
Carbs

30g

105
Cals

4g
Prot

10g
Fat

3g
SatFat

0g
Fibre

BBQ Ribs

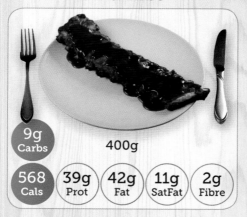

9g Carbs

400g

568 Cals

39g Prot

42g Fat

11g SatFat

2g Fibre

Gammon (grilled)

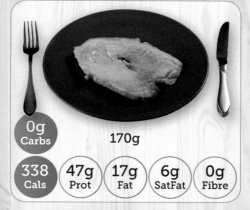

0g Carbs

170g

338 Cals

47g Prot

17g Fat

6g SatFat

0g Fibre

Pork Chop (grilled)

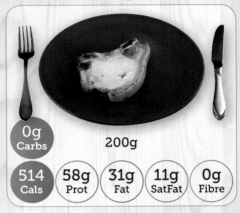

0g Carbs

200g

514 Cals | 58g Prot | 31g Fat | 11g SatFat | 0g Fibre

Roast Pork

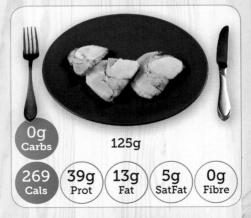

0g Carbs

125g

269 Cals | 39g Prot | 13g Fat | 5g SatFat | 0g Fibre

Back Bacon (fried)

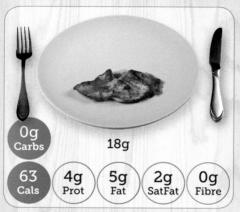

0g
Carbs

18g

63
Cals

4g
Prot

5g
Fat

2g
SatFat

0g
Fibre

Back Bacon (grilled)

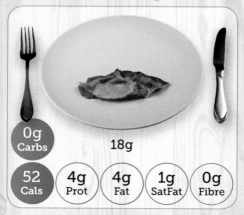

0g
Carbs

18g

52
Cals

4g
Prot

4g
Fat

1g
SatFat

0g
Fibre

Streaky Bacon (fried)

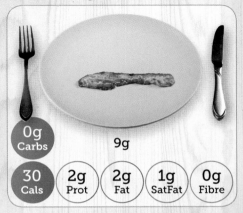

0g
Carbs

9g

30
Cals

2g
Prot

2g
Fat

1g
SatFat

0g
Fibre

Streaky Bacon (grilled)

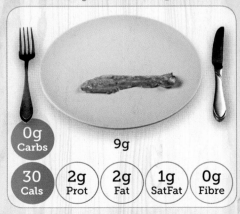

0g
Carbs

9g

30
Cals

2g
Prot

2g
Fat

1g
SatFat

0g
Fibre

Sausage (grilled)

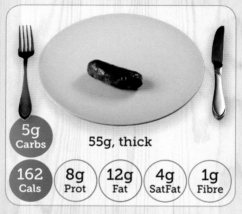

5g Carbs

55g, thick

162 Cals · **8g** Prot · **12g** Fat · **4g** SatFat · **1g** Fibre

Chorizo

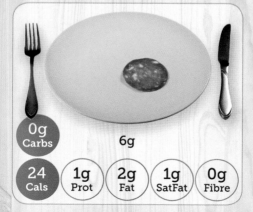

0g Carbs

6g

24 Cals · **1g** Prot · **2g** Fat · **1g** SatFat · **0g** Fibre

Pancetta (dry fried)

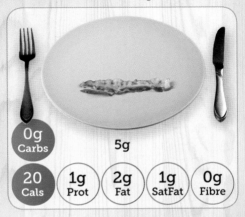

0g Carbs

5g

20 Cals

1g Prot

2g Fat

1g SatFat

0g Fibre

Parma Ham

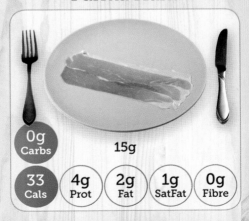

0g Carbs

15g

33 Cals

4g Prot

2g Fat

1g SatFat

0g Fibre

Prosciutto

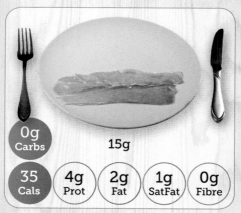

0g Carbs

15g

35 Cals

4g Prot

2g Fat

1g SatFat

0g Fibre

Salami

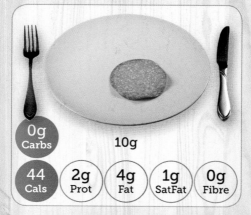

0g Carbs

10g

44 Cals

2g Prot

4g Fat

1g SatFat

0g Fibre

Beef Slice

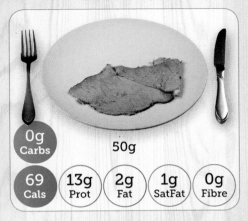

0g Carbs

50g

69 Cals

13g Prot

2g Fat

1g SatFat

0g Fibre

Wafer-thin Beef

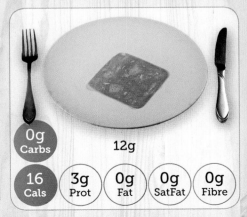

0g Carbs

12g

16 Cals

3g Prot

0g Fat

0g SatFat

0g Fibre

Ham Slice

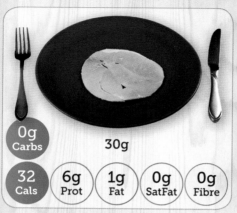

0g Carbs

30g

32 Cals

6g Prot

1g Fat

0g SatFat

0g Fibre

Wafer-thin Ham

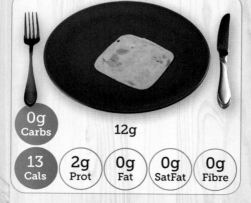

0g Carbs

12g

13 Cals

2g Prot

0g Fat

0g SatFat

0g Fibre

Turkey Slice

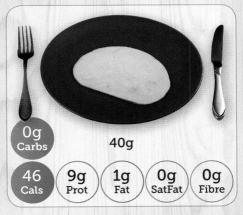

0g
Carbs

40g

46
Cals

9g
Prot

1g
Fat

0g
SatFat

0g
Fibre

Wafer-thin Turkey

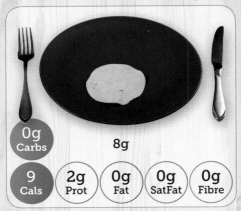

0g
Carbs

8g

9
Cals

2g
Prot

0g
Fat

0g
SatFat

0g
Fibre

Beef Burger (fried)

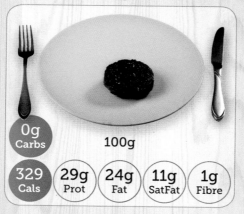

0g Carbs

100g

329 Cals | 29g Prot | 24g Fat | 11g SatFat | 1g Fibre

Beef Burger (grilled)

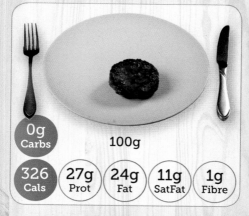

0g Carbs

100g

326 Cals | 27g Prot | 24g Fat | 11g SatFat | 1g Fibre

Corned Beef

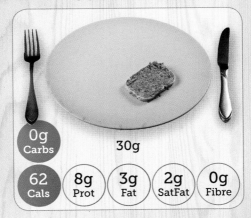

0g Carbs

30g

62 Cals | **8g** Prot | **3g** Fat | **2g** SatFat | **0g** Fibre

Roast Beef

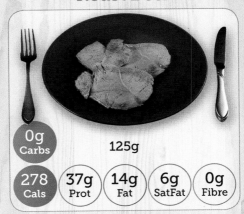

0g Carbs

125g

278 Cals | **37g** Prot | **14g** Fat | **6g** SatFat | **0g** Fibre

Rump Steak (fried)

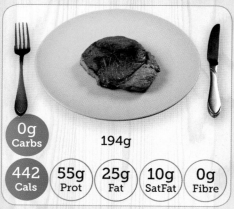

0g
Carbs

194g

442
Cals

55g
Prot

25g
Fat

10g
SatFat

0g
Fibre

Sirloin Steak (fried)

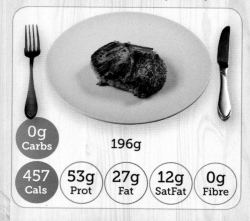

0g
Carbs

196g

457
Cals

53g
Prot

27g
Fat

12g
SatFat

0g
Fibre

Lamb Chop (grilled)

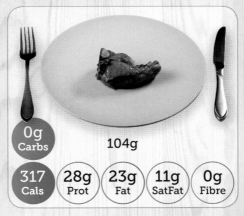

0g Carbs

104g

317 Cals | **28g** Prot | **23g** Fat | **11g** SatFat | **0g** Fibre

Lamb Steak (grilled)

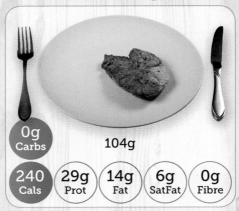

0g Carbs

104g

240 Cals | **29g** Prot | **14g** Fat | **6g** SatFat | **0g** Fibre

Roast Lamb

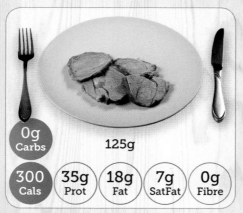

0g Carbs

125g

300 Cals | **35g** Prot | **18g** Fat | **7g** SatFat | **0g** Fibre

Wafer-thin Chicken

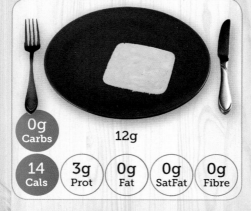

0g Carbs

12g

14 Cals | **3g** Prot | **0g** Fat | **0g** SatFat | **0g** Fibre

BBQ Chicken Wings

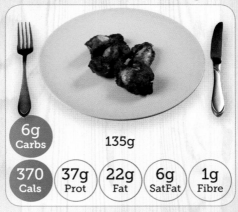

6g Carbs

135g

370 Cals | **37g** Prot | **22g** Fat | **6g** SatFat | **1g** Fibre

Chicken Drumstick (roasted)

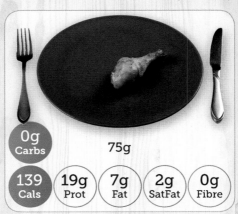

0g Carbs

75g

139 Cals | **19g** Prot | **7g** Fat | **2g** SatFat | **0g** Fibre

Chicken Breast
(grilled, without skin)

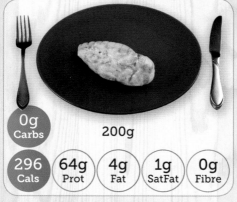

0g
Carbs

200g

296
Cals

64g
Prot

4g
Fat

1g
SatFat

0g
Fibre

Chicken Breast
(grilled, with skin)

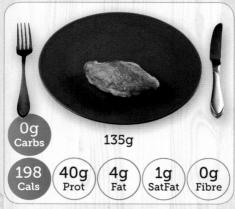

0g
Carbs

135g

198
Cals

40g
Prot

4g
Fat

1g
SatFat

0g
Fibre

Roast Chicken (with skin)

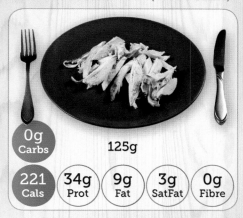

0g Carbs

125g

221 Cals | **34g** Prot | **9g** Fat | **3g** SatFat | **0g** Fibre

Chicken Kiev

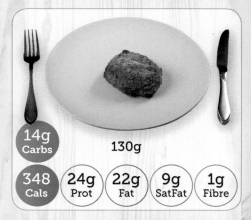

14g Carbs

130g

348 Cals | **24g** Prot | **22g** Fat | **9g** SatFat | **1g** Fibre

Roast Turkey (with skin)

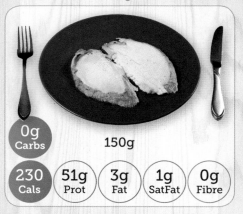

0g Carbs

150g

230 Cals | 51g Prot | 3g Fat | 1g SatFat | 0g Fibre

Turkey Breast (grilled)

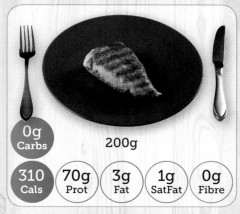

0g Carbs

200g

310 Cals | 70g Prot | 3g Fat | 1g SatFat | 0g Fibre

Fish (battered, baked)

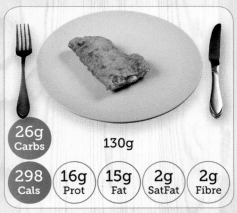

26g Carbs

130g

298 Cals | **16g Prot** | **15g Fat** | **2g SatFat** | **2g Fibre**

Fish (breaded, baked)

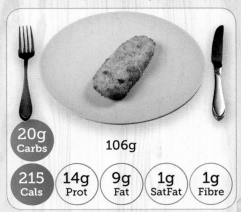

20g Carbs

106g

215 Cals | **14g Prot** | **9g Fat** | **1g SatFat** | **1g Fibre**

Fish Cake (baked)

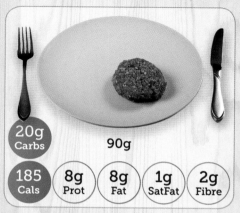

20g
Carbs

90g

185
Cals

8g
Prot

8g
Fat

1g
SatFat

2g
Fibre

Fish Finger (baked)

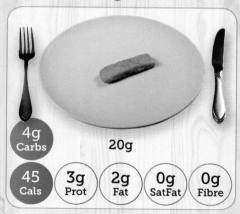

4g
Carbs

20g

45
Cals

3g
Prot

2g
Fat

0g
SatFat

0g
Fibre

Fish Goujon (baked)

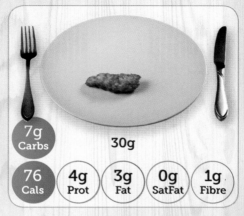

7g
Carbs

30g

76
Cals

4g
Prot

3g
Fat

0g
SatFat

1g
Fibre

Scampi (fried)

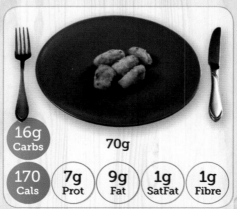

16g
Carbs

70g

170
Cals

7g
Prot

9g
Fat

1g
SatFat

1g
Fibre

Prawns (boiled)

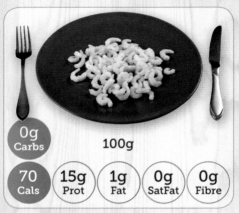

0g Carbs

100g

70 Cals | 15g Prot | 1g Fat | 0g SatFat | 0g Fibre

King Prawns (boiled)

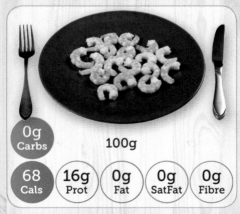

0g Carbs

100g

68 Cals | 16g Prot | 0g Fat | 0g SatFat | 0g Fibre

Salmon (tinned in brine)

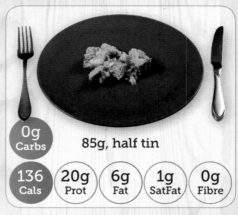

0g Carbs

85g, half tin

136 Cals | **20g** Prot | **6g** Fat | **1g** SatFat | **0g** Fibre

Tuna (tinned in brine)

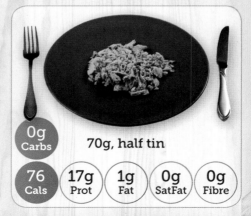

0g Carbs

70g, half tin

76 Cals | **17g** Prot | **1g** Fat | **0g** SatFat | **0g** Fibre

Tuna (tinned in oil)

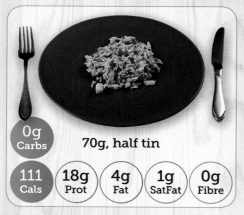

0g Carbs

70g, half tin

111 Cals   **18g** Prot   **4g** Fat   **1g** SatFat   **0g** Fibre

Sardines (tinned in brine)

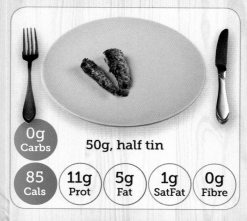

0g Carbs

50g, half tin

85 Cals   **11g** Prot   **5g** Fat   **1g** SatFat   **0g** Fibre

Sardines (tinned in oil)

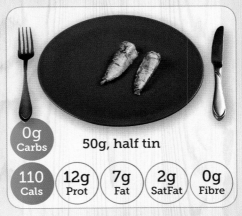

0g Carbs

50g, half tin

110 Cals | **12g** Prot | **7g** Fat | **2g** SatFat | **0g** Fibre

Sardines
(tinned in tomato sauce)

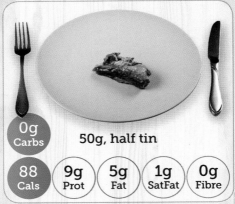

0g Carbs

50g, half tin

88 Cals | **9g** Prot | **5g** Fat | **1g** SatFat | **0g** Fibre

Smoked Mackerel

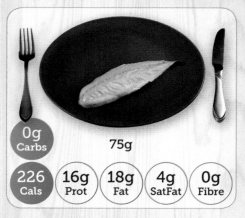

0g
Carbs

75g

226
Cals

16g
Prot

18g
Fat

4g
SatFat

0g
Fibre

Smoked Salmon

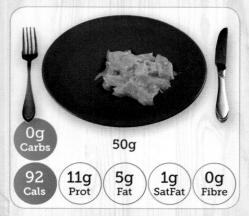

0g
Carbs

50g

92
Cals

11g
Prot

5g
Fat

1g
SatFat

0g
Fibre

Saltfish (boiled)

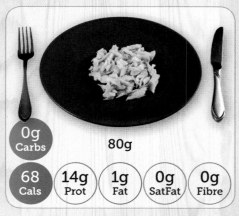

0g Carbs

80g

68 Cals | **14g** Prot | **1g** Fat | **0g** SatFat | **0g** Fibre

Cod / Haddock (baked)

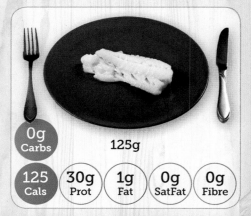

0g Carbs

125g

125 Cals | **30g** Prot | **1g** Fat | **0g** SatFat | **0g** Fibre

Plaice (grilled)

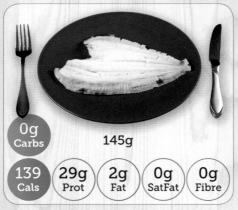

0g
Carbs

145g

139
Cals

29g
Prot

2g
Fat

0g
SatFat

0g
Fibre

Scallops (fried)

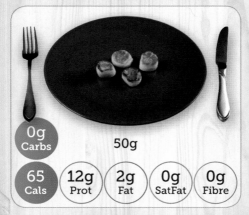

0g
Carbs

50g

65
Cals

12g
Prot

2g
Fat

0g
SatFat

0g
Fibre

Salmon Steak (grilled)

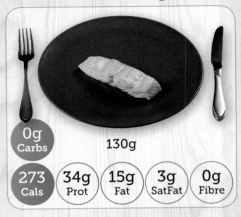

0g Carbs

130g

273 Cals | **34g** Prot | **15g** Fat | **3g** SatFat | **0g** Fibre

Trout Fillet (baked)

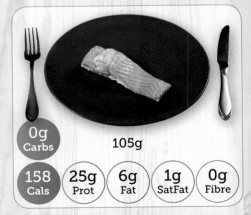

0g Carbs

105g

158 Cals | **25g** Prot | **6g** Fat | **1g** SatFat | **0g** Fibre

Tuna Steak (grilled)

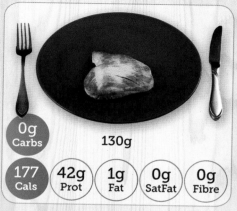

0g Carbs

130g

177 Cals | **42g** Prot | **1g** Fat | **0g** SatFat | **0g** Fibre

Crab Meat (tinned)

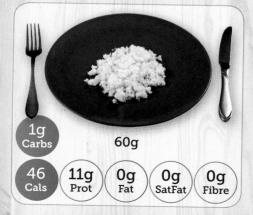

1g Carbs

60g

46 Cals | **11g** Prot | **0g** Fat | **0g** SatFat | **0g** Fibre

Seafood Sticks

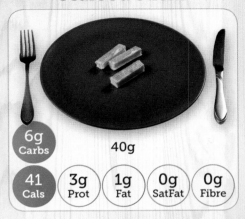

6g Carbs

40g

41 Cals | 3g Prot | 1g Fat | 0g SatFat | 0g Fibre

Calamari (fried)

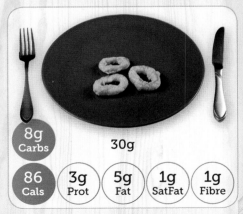

8g Carbs

30g

86 Cals | 3g Prot | 5g Fat | 1g SatFat | 1g Fibre

Almond Milk

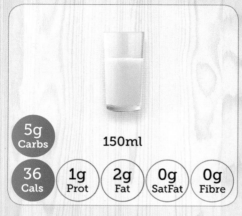

5g Carbs

150ml

36 Cals — **1g** Prot — **2g** Fat — **0g** SatFat — **0g** Fibre

Coconut Milk

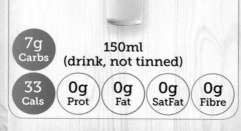

7g Carbs

150ml
(drink, not tinned)

33 Cals — **0g** Prot — **0g** Fat — **0g** SatFat — **0g** Fibre

Goat's Milk

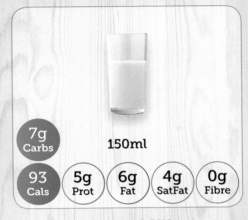

7g Carbs

150ml

93 Cals | **5g** Prot | **6g** Fat | **4g** SatFat | **0g** Fibre

Hemp Milk

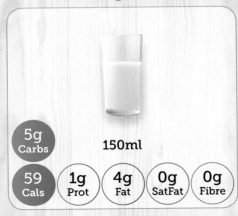

5g Carbs

150ml

59 Cals | **1g** Prot | **4g** Fat | **0g** SatFat | **0g** Fibre

Oat Milk

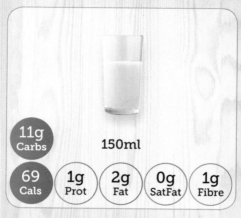

11g Carbs

150ml

69 Cals

1g Prot

2g Fat

0g SatFat

1g Fibre

Rice Milk

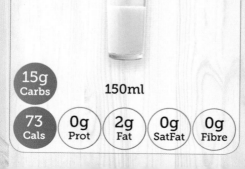

15g Carbs

150ml

73 Cals

0g Prot

2g Fat

0g SatFat

0g Fibre

Milk (whole)

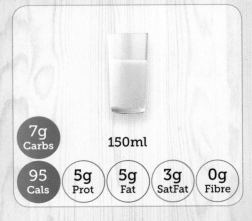

7g Carbs

150ml

95 Cals | **5g** Prot | **5g** Fat | **3g** SatFat | **0g** Fibre

Milk (semi-skimmed)

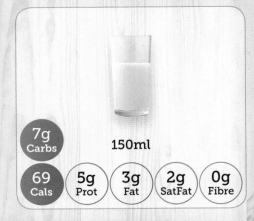

7g Carbs

150ml

69 Cals | **5g** Prot | **3g** Fat | **2g** SatFat | **0g** Fibre

Milk (1%)

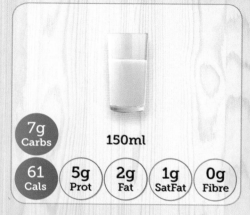

7g Carbs

150ml

61 Cals | **5g** Prot | **2g** Fat | **1g** SatFat | **0g** Fibre

Milk (skimmed)

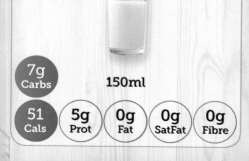

7g Carbs

150ml

51 Cals | **5g** Prot | **0g** Fat | **0g** SatFat | **0g** Fibre

Soya Milk (sweetened)

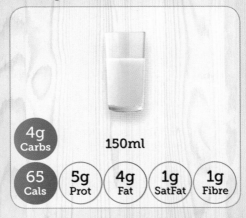

4g Carbs

150ml

65 Cals   **5g** Prot   **4g** Fat   **1g** SatFat   **1g** Fibre

Soya Milk (unsweetened)

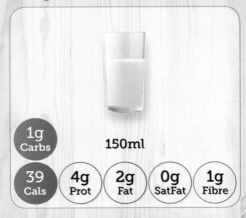

1g Carbs

150ml

39 Cals   **4g** Prot   **2g** Fat   **0g** SatFat   **1g** Fibre

Milkshake
(powder & semi-skimmed milk)

33g Carbs

284ml, half pint
(chocolate)

203 Cals | **9g** Prot | **4g** Fat | **3g** SatFat | **0g** Fibre

Milkshake
(powder & semi-skimmed milk)

29g Carbs

284ml, half pint
(strawberry)

196 Cals | **9g** Prot | **5g** Fat | **3g** SatFat | **0g** Fibre

Single Cream

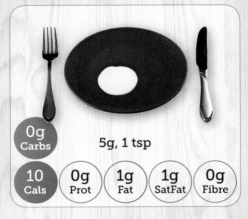

0g Carbs

5g, 1 tsp

10 Cals | 0g Prot | 1g Fat | 1g SatFat | 0g Fibre

Double Cream

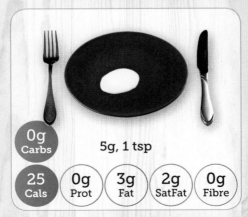

0g Carbs

5g, 1 tsp

25 Cals | 0g Prot | 3g Fat | 2g SatFat | 0g Fibre

Clotted Cream

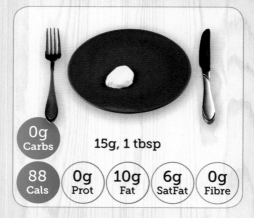

0g Carbs

15g, 1 tbsp

88 Cals

0g Prot

10g Fat

6g SatFat

0g Fibre

Crème Fraîche

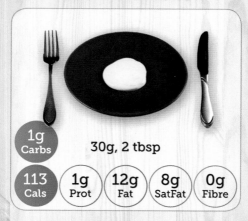

1g Carbs

30g, 2 tbsp

113 Cals

1g Prot

12g Fat

8g SatFat

0g Fibre

Soured Cream

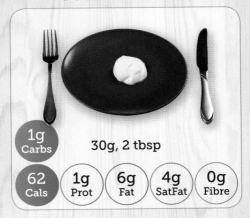

1g Carbs

30g, 2 tbsp

62 Cals | **1g** Prot | **6g** Fat | **4g** SatFat | **0g** Fibre

Whipped Cream

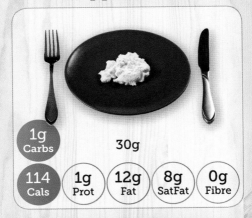

1g Carbs

30g

114 Cals | **1g** Prot | **12g** Fat | **8g** SatFat | **0g** Fibre

Almonds

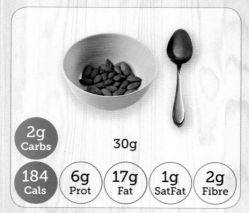

2g Carbs

30g

184 Cals

6g Prot

17g Fat

1g SatFat

2g Fibre

Brazil Nuts

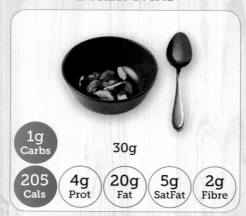

1g Carbs

30g

205 Cals

4g Prot

20g Fat

5g SatFat

2g Fibre

Cashews

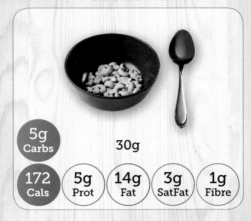

5g Carbs

30g

172 Cals | 5g Prot | 14g Fat | 3g SatFat | 1g Fibre

Dried Fruit & Nuts

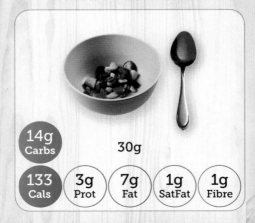

14g Carbs

30g

133 Cals | 3g Prot | 7g Fat | 1g SatFat | 1g Fibre

Hazelnuts

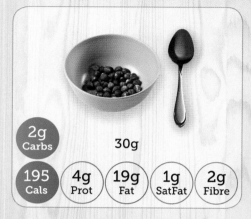

2g Carbs

30g

195 Cals | **4g** Prot | **19g** Fat | **1g** SatFat | **2g** Fibre

Macadamia Nuts

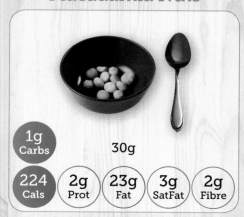

1g Carbs

30g

224 Cals | **2g** Prot | **23g** Fat | **3g** SatFat | **2g** Fibre

Peanuts (roasted)

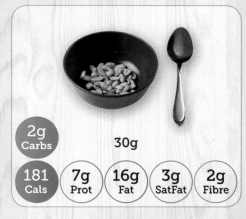

2g
Carbs

30g

181
Cals

7g
Prot

16g
Fat

3g
SatFat

2g
Fibre

Pecans

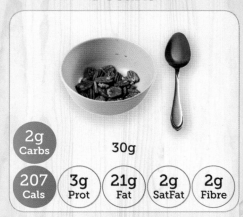

2g
Carbs

30g

207
Cals

3g
Prot

21g
Fat

2g
SatFat

2g
Fibre

Pistachios

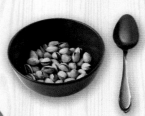

2g Carbs

60g, with shells

180 Cals   **5g** Prot   **17g** Fat   **2g** SatFat   **2g** Fibre

Pistachios

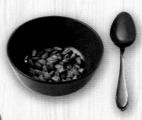

2g Carbs

30g, without shells

180 Cals   **5g** Prot   **17g** Fat   **2g** SatFat   **2g** Fibre

Pine Nuts

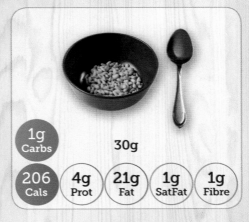

1g Carbs

30g

206 Cals

4g Prot

21g Fat

1g SatFat

1g Fibre

Soya Nuts

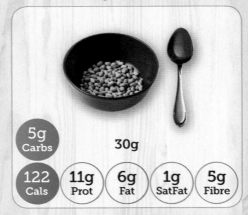

5g Carbs

30g

122 Cals

11g Prot

6g Fat

1g SatFat

5g Fibre

Walnuts

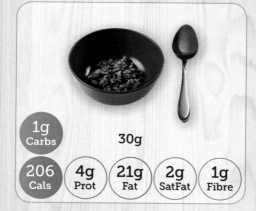

1g Carbs

30g

206 Cals

4g Prot

21g Fat

2g SatFat

1g Fibre

Linseeds / Flaxseeds

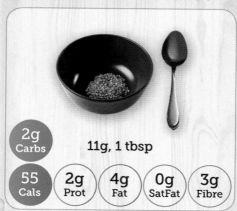

2g Carbs

11g, 1 tbsp

55 Cals

2g Prot

4g Fat

0g SatFat

3g Fibre

Pumpkin Seeds

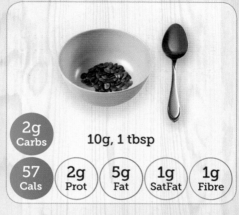

2g Carbs

10g, 1 tbsp

57 Cals

2g Prot

5g Fat

1g SatFat

1g Fibre

Sunflower Seeds

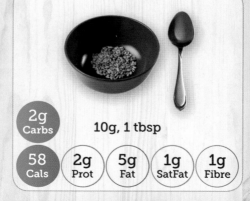

2g Carbs

10g, 1 tbsp

58 Cals

2g Prot

5g Fat

1g SatFat

1g Fibre

Macaroni

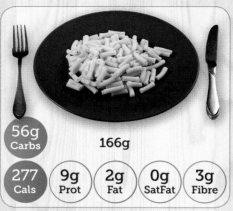

56g Carbs

166g

277 Cals

9g Prot

2g Fat

0g SatFat

3g Fibre

Pasta Shells

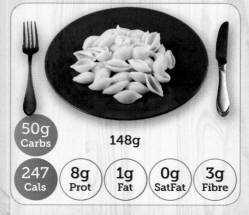

50g Carbs

148g

247 Cals

8g Prot

1g Fat

0g SatFat

3g Fibre

Pasta Twists

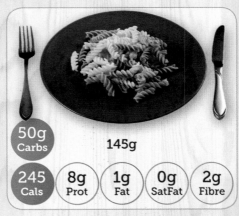

50g Carbs

145g

245 Cals | **8g** Prot | **1g** Fat | **0g** SatFat | **2g** Fibre

Penne

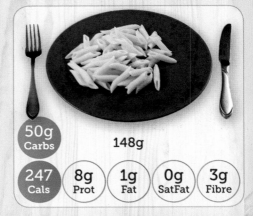

50g Carbs

148g

247 Cals | **8g** Prot | **1g** Fat | **0g** SatFat | **3g** Fibre

Ravioli (fresh, meat-filled)

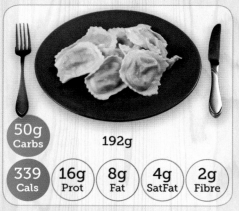

50g Carbs

192g

339 Cals | **16g** Prot | **8g** Fat | **4g** SatFat | **2g** Fibre

Spaghetti (white)

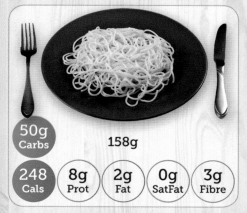

50g Carbs

158g

248 Cals | **8g** Prot | **2g** Fat | **0g** SatFat | **3g** Fibre

Spaghetti (whole wheat)

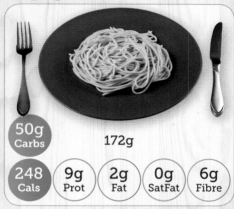

50g Carbs

172g

248 Cals

| 9g Prot | 2g Fat | 0g SatFat | 6g Fibre |

Tagliatelle

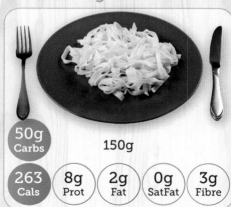

50g Carbs

150g

263 Cals

| 8g Prot | 2g Fat | 0g SatFat | 3g Fibre |

Tortellini (fresh, cheese-filled)

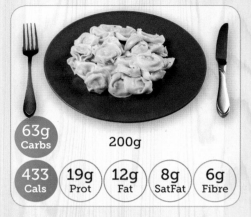

63g Carbs

200g

433 Cals

| 19g Prot | 12g Fat | 8g SatFat | 6g Fibre |

Vermicelli

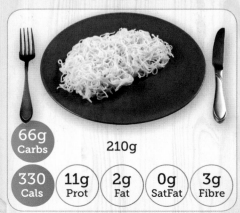

66g Carbs

210g

330 Cals

| 11g Prot | 2g Fat | 0g SatFat | 3g Fibre |

Noodles (egg)

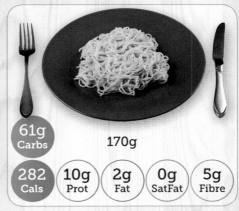

61g Carbs

170g

282 Cals

10g Prot

2g Fat

0g SatFat

5g Fibre

Noodles (rice)

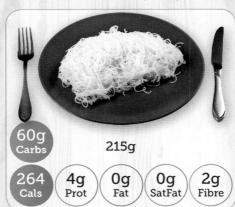

60g Carbs

215g

264 Cals

4g Prot

0g Fat

0g SatFat

2g Fibre

Pasta Shapes (tinned)

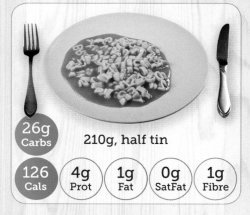

26g Carbs

210g, half tin

126 Cals

4g Prot

1g Fat

0g SatFat

1g Fibre

Ravioli (tinned)

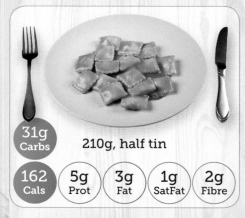

31g Carbs

210g, half tin

162 Cals

5g Prot

3g Fat

1g SatFat

2g Fibre

Spaghetti (tinned)

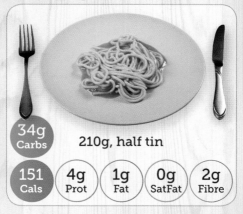

34g Carbs

210g, half tin

151 Cals

4g Prot

1g Fat

0g SatFat

2g Fibre

Spaghetti Hoops (tinned)

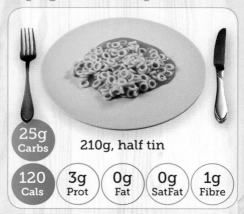

25g Carbs

210g, half tin

120 Cals

3g Prot

0g Fat

0g SatFat

1g Fibre

Chips (deep fried)

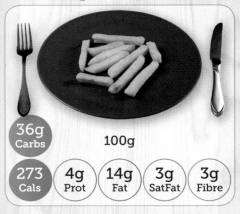

36g Carbs

100g

273 Cals

4g Prot

14g Fat

3g SatFat

3g Fibre

Chips (oven)

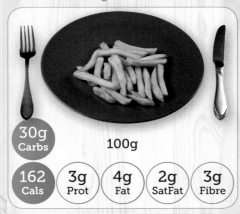

30g Carbs

100g

162 Cals

3g Prot

4g Fat

2g SatFat

3g Fibre

Dauphinoise Potatoes

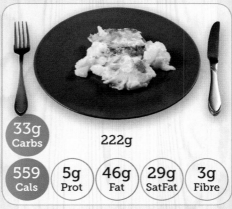

33g Carbs

222g

559 Cals

5g Prot

46g Fat

29g SatFat

3g Fibre

Gnocchi

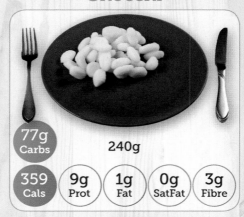

77g Carbs

240g

359 Cals

9g Prot

1g Fat

0g SatFat

3g Fibre

Jacket Potato (baked)

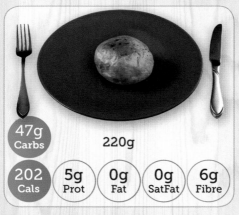

47g Carbs

220g

202 Cals

5g Prot

0g Fat

0g SatFat

6g Fibre

New Potatoes (boiled)

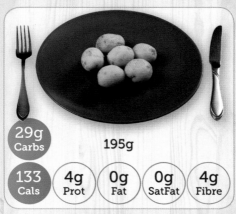

29g Carbs

195g

133 Cals

4g Prot

0g Fat

0g SatFat

4g Fibre

Mashed Potato
(with semi-skimmed milk)

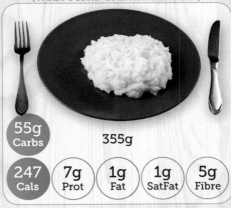

55g Carbs

355g

247 Cals | **7g** Prot | **1g** Fat | **1g** SatFat | **5g** Fibre

Potato Slices (baked)

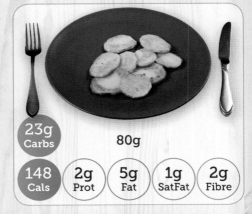

23g Carbs

80g

148 Cals | **2g** Prot | **5g** Fat | **1g** SatFat | **2g** Fibre

Roast Potatoes (in oil)

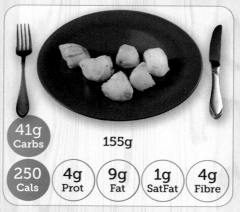

41g Carbs

155g

250 Cals

4g Prot

9g Fat

1g SatFat

4g Fibre

Sweet Potatoes (baked)

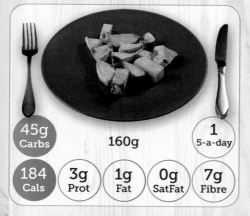

45g Carbs

160g

1 5-a-day

184 Cals

3g Prot

1g Fat

0g SatFat

7g Fibre

Mashed Sweet Potato

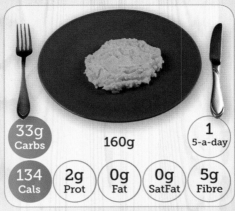

33g Carbs

160g

1 5-a-day

134 Cals

2g Prot

0g Fat

0g SatFat

5g Fibre

Potato Salad
(with mayonnaise)

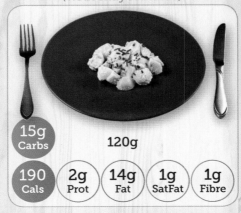

15g Carbs

120g

190 Cals

2g Prot

14g Fat

1g SatFat

1g Fibre

Wedges (baked)

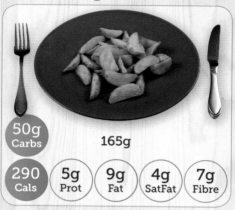

50g Carbs

165g

290 Cals

5g Prot

9g Fat

4g SatFat

7g Fibre

Hash Brown (baked)

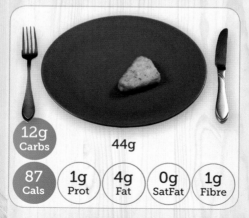

12g Carbs

44g

87 Cals

1g Prot

4g Fat

0g SatFat

1g Fibre

Potato Croquette (fried)

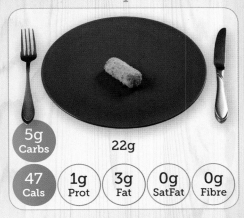

5g Carbs

22g

47 Cals

1g Prot

3g Fat

0g SatFat

0g Fibre

Potato Rosti (grilled)

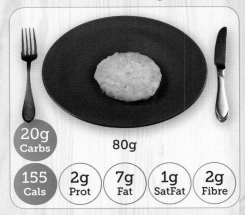

20g Carbs

80g

155 Cals

2g Prot

7g Fat

1g SatFat

2g Fibre

Potato Waffle (baked)

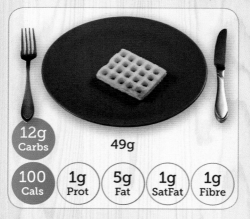

12g Carbs

49g

100 Cals | **1g** Prot | **5g** Fat | **1g** SatFat | **1g** Fibre

Potato Smiles (baked)

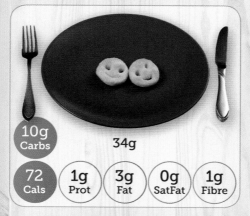

10g Carbs

34g

72 Cals | **1g** Prot | **3g** Fat | **0g** SatFat | **1g** Fibre

Cassava Chips (baked)

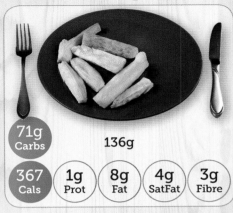

71g Carbs

136g

367 Cals

1g Prot	8g Fat	4g SatFat	3g Fibre

Eba / Gari

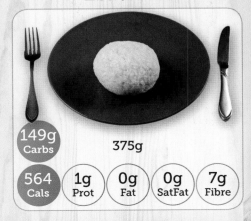

149g Carbs

375g

564 Cals

1g Prot	0g Fat	0g SatFat	7g Fibre

Fufu (plantain)

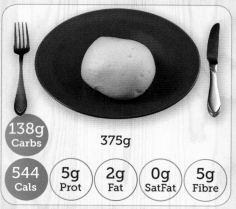

138g
Carbs

375g

544
Cals

5g
Prot

2g
Fat

0g
SatFat

5g
Fibre

Yam (boiled)

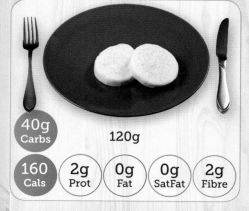

40g
Carbs

120g

160
Cals

2g
Prot

0g
Fat

0g
SatFat

2g
Fibre

Basmati Rice

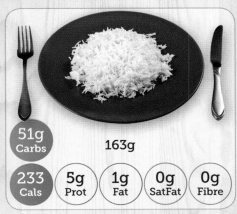

51g
Carbs

163g

233
Cals

5g
Prot

1g
Fat

0g
SatFat

0g
Fibre

Brown Rice (wholegrain)

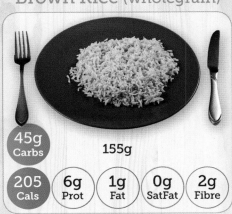

45g
Carbs

155g

205
Cals

6g
Prot

1g
Fat

0g
SatFat

2g
Fibre

White Rice (long grain)

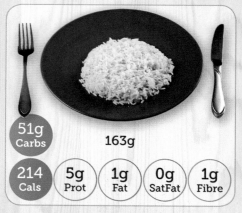

51g Carbs

163g

214 Cals | **5g** Prot | **1g** Fat | **0g** SatFat | **1g** Fibre

Egg Fried Rice

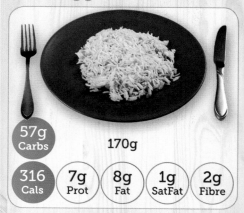

57g Carbs

170g

316 Cals | **7g** Prot | **8g** Fat | **1g** SatFat | **2g** Fibre

Jollof Rice

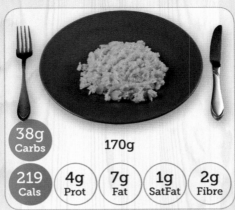

38g Carbs

170g

219 Cals | **4g** Prot | **7g** Fat | **1g** SatFat | **2g** Fibre

Mexican Rice

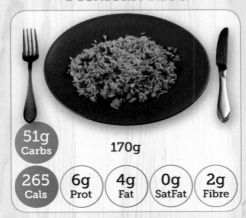

51g Carbs

170g

265 Cals | **6g** Prot | **4g** Fat | **0g** SatFat | **2g** Fibre

Pilau Rice

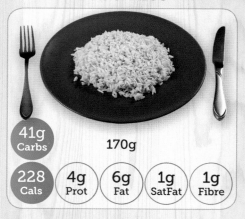

41g Carbs

170g

228 Cals

4g Prot

6g Fat

1g SatFat

1g Fibre

Rice & Peas

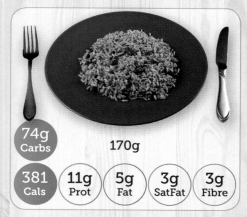

74g Carbs

170g

381 Cals

11g Prot

5g Fat

3g SatFat

3g Fibre

Special Fried Rice

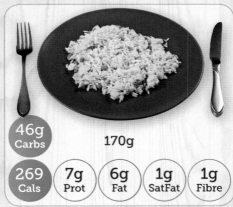

46g Carbs

170g

269 Cals

7g Prot

6g Fat

1g SatFat

1g Fibre

Sticky White Rice

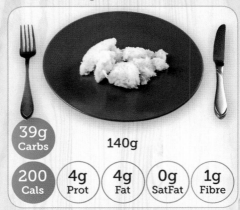

39g Carbs

140g

200 Cals

4g Prot

4g Fat

0g SatFat

1g Fibre

Wild Rice

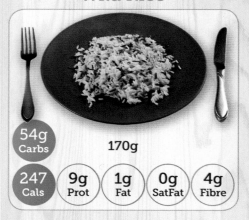

54g Carbs

170g

247 Cals · **9g** Prot · **1g** Fat · **0g** SatFat · **4g** Fibre

Bulgur Wheat

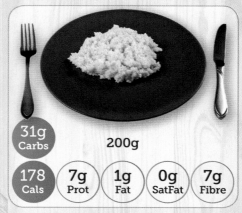

31g Carbs

200g

178 Cals · **7g** Prot · **1g** Fat · **0g** SatFat · **7g** Fibre

Couscous

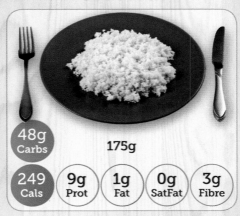

48g Carbs

175g

249 Cals | **9g** Prot | **1g** Fat | **0g** SatFat | **3g** Fibre

Quinoa

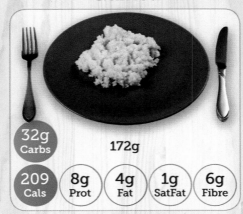

32g Carbs

172g

209 Cals | **8g** Prot | **4g** Fat | **1g** SatFat | **6g** Fibre

Polenta

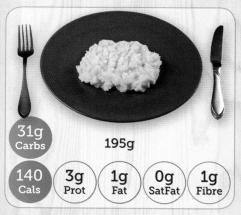

31g Carbs

195g

140 Cals

3g Prot

1g Fat

0g SatFat

1g Fibre

Polenta (sliced)

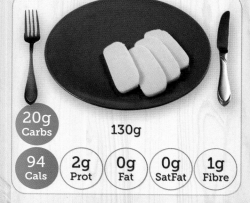

20g Carbs

130g

94 Cals

2g Prot

0g Fat

0g SatFat

1g Fibre

BLT

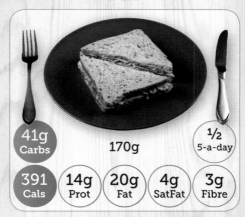

41g Carbs

170g

½ 5-a-day

391 Cals

14g Prot

20g Fat

4g SatFat

3g Fibre

Cheese & Pickle

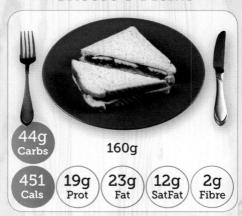

44g Carbs

160g

451 Cals

19g Prot

23g Fat

12g SatFat

2g Fibre

Chicken Salad

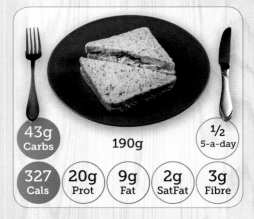

43g Carbs

190g

½ 5-a-day

327 Cals

20g Prot

9g Fat

2g SatFat

3g Fibre

Coronation Chicken

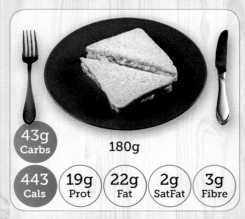

43g Carbs

180g

443 Cals

19g Prot

22g Fat

2g SatFat

3g Fibre

Egg Mayo

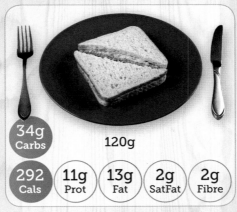

34g Carbs

120g

292 Cals | **11g** Prot | **13g** Fat | **2g** SatFat | **2g** Fibre

Ham Salad

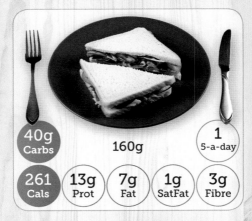

40g Carbs

160g

1 5-a-day

261 Cals | **13g** Prot | **7g** Fat | **1g** SatFat | **3g** Fibre

Prawn Mayo

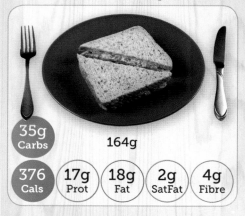

35g Carbs

164g

376 Cals

17g Prot

18g Fat

2g SatFat

4g Fibre

Tuna Mayo & Sweetcorn

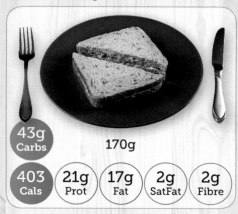

43g Carbs

170g

403 Cals

21g Prot

17g Fat

2g SatFat

2g Fibre

Bombay Mix

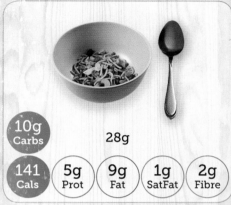

10g
Carbs

28g

141
Cals

5g
Prot

9g
Fat

1g
SatFat

2g
Fibre

Crisps

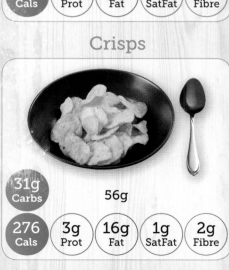

31g
Carbs

56g

276
Cals

3g
Prot

16g
Fat

1g
SatFat

2g
Fibre

Popcorn (salted)

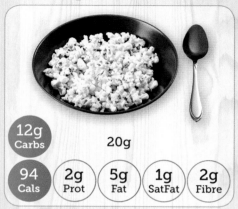

12g Carbs

20g

94 Cals | **2g** Prot | **5g** Fat | **1g** SatFat | **2g** Fibre

Popcorn (sweet)

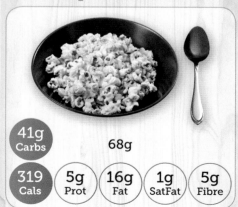

41g Carbs

68g

319 Cals | **5g** Prot | **16g** Fat | **1g** SatFat | **5g** Fibre

Pretzels

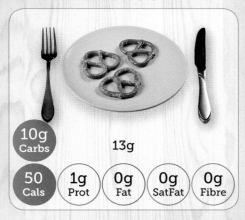

10g Carbs

13g

50 Cals | **1g Prot** | **0g Fat** | **0g SatFat** | **0g Fibre**

Tortilla Chips

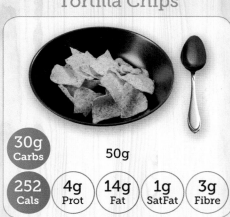

30g Carbs

50g

252 Cals | **4g Prot** | **14g Fat** | **1g SatFat** | **3g Fibre**

Fudge

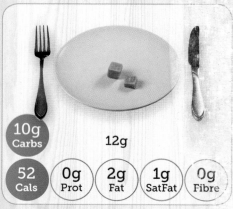

10g Carbs

12g

52 Cals

0g Prot

2g Fat

1g SatFat

0g Fibre

Marshmallows (small)

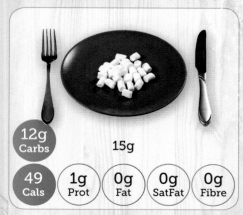

12g Carbs

15g

49 Cals

1g Prot

0g Fat

0g SatFat

0g Fibre

Marshmallows (large)

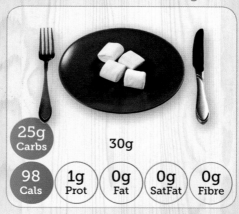

25g Carbs

30g

98 Cals | **1g** Prot | **0g** Fat | **0g** SatFat | **0g** Fibre

Chocolate (milk)

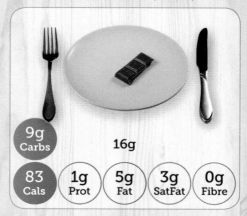

9g Carbs

16g

83 Cals | **1g** Prot | **5g** Fat | **3g** SatFat | **0g** Fibre

Chocolate (dark)

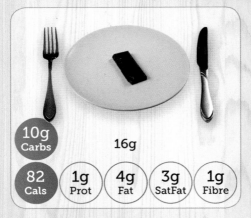

10g Carbs

16g

82 Cals | 1g Prot | 4g Fat | 3g SatFat | 1g Fibre

Chocolate (white)

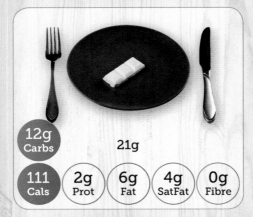

12g Carbs

21g

111 Cals | 2g Prot | 6g Fat | 4g SatFat | 0g Fibre

Chocolate
(milk, with hazelnuts)

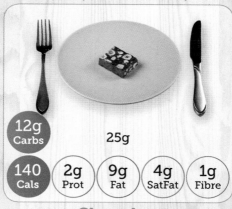

12g Carbs

25g

140 Cals

2g Prot

9g Fat

4g SatFat

1g Fibre

Chocolate
Honeycomb Balls

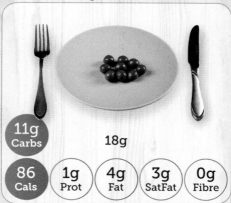

11g Carbs

18g

86 Cals

1g Prot

4g Fat

3g SatFat

0g Fibre

Chocolate Mint

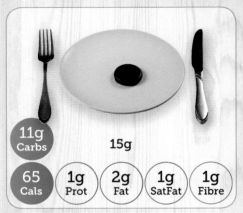

11g
Carbs

15g

65
Cals

1g
Prot

2g
Fat

1g
SatFat

1g
Fibre

Individual Chocolate

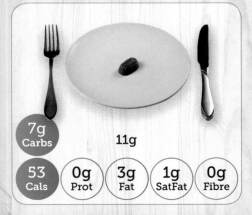

7g
Carbs

11g

53
Cals

0g
Prot

3g
Fat

1g
SatFat

0g
Fibre

Individual Chocolate

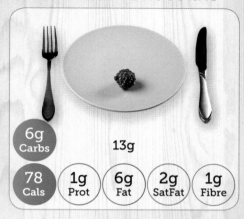

6g
Carbs

13g

78
Cals

1g
Prot

6g
Fat

2g
SatFat

1g
Fibre

Chocolate Orange

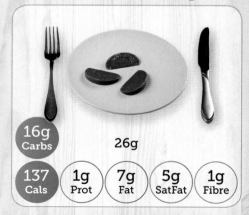

16g
Carbs

26g

137
Cals

1g
Prot

7g
Fat

5g
SatFat

1g
Fibre

Chocolate Bunny

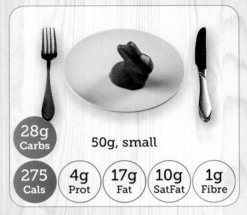

28g Carbs

50g, small

275 Cals

4g Prot

17g Fat

10g SatFat

1g Fibre

Easter Egg

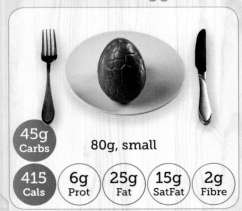

45g Carbs

80g, small

415 Cals

6g Prot

25g Fat

15g SatFat

2g Fibre

Easter Egg

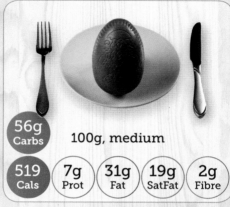

56g Carbs

100g, medium

519 Cals

7g Prot

31g Fat

19g SatFat

2g Fibre

Easter Egg

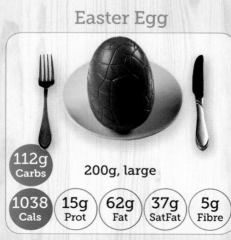

112g Carbs

200g, large

1038 Cals

15g Prot

62g Fat

37g SatFat

5g Fibre

Mini Eggs

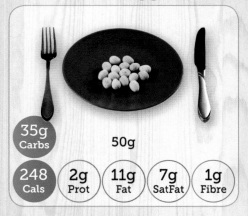

35g Carbs

50g

248 Cals

2g Prot

11g Fat

7g SatFat

1g Fibre

Alpen Bar
(Raspberry & Yogurt)

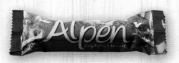

22g Carbs

29g

123 Cals

1g Prot

3g Fat

2g SatFat

1g Fibre

Alpen Bar Light
(Double Chocolate)

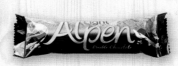

12g Carbs

21g

72 Cals | **1g** Prot | **1g** Fat | **1g** SatFat | **0g** Fibre

Nakd Bar (Berry Delight)

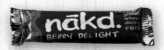

18g Carbs

35g

1 5-a-day

135 Cals | **3g** Prot | **5g** Fat | **1g** SatFat | **2g** Fibre

Cola Bottles

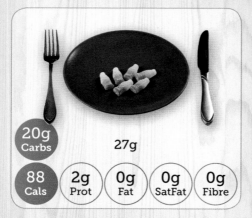

20g
Carbs

27g

88 Cals

2g Prot

0g Fat

0g SatFat

0g Fibre

Dextrose Tablets

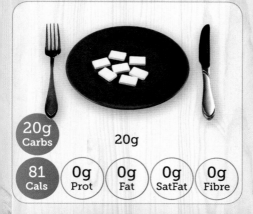

20g
Carbs

20g

81 Cals

0g Prot

0g Fat

0g SatFat

0g Fibre

Jelly Babies

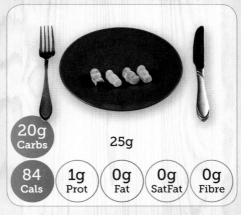

20g Carbs

25g

84 Cals

1g Prot

0g Fat

0g SatFat

0g Fibre

Jelly Beans

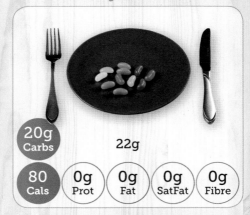

20g Carbs

22g

80 Cals

0g Prot

0g Fat

0g SatFat

0g Fibre

Licorice Allsorts

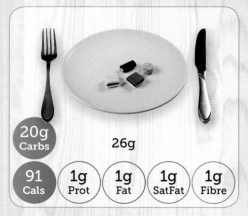

20g Carbs

26g

91 Cals

1g Prot

1g Fat

1g SatFat

1g Fibre

Wine Gums

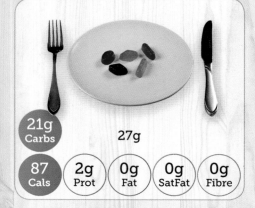

21g Carbs

27g

87 Cals

2g Prot

0g Fat

0g SatFat

0g Fibre

Broccoli & Stilton Soup

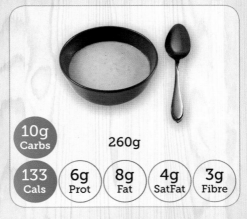

10g Carbs

260g

133 Cals

6g Prot

8g Fat

4g SatFat

3g Fibre

Chicken Noodle Soup

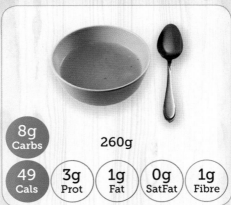

8g Carbs

260g

49 Cals

3g Prot

1g Fat

0g SatFat

1g Fibre

Chunky Veg Soup

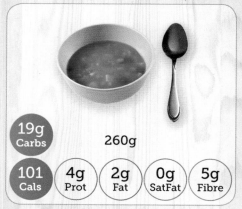

19g Carbs

260g

101 Cals

4g Prot

2g Fat

0g SatFat

5g Fibre

Mushroom Soup

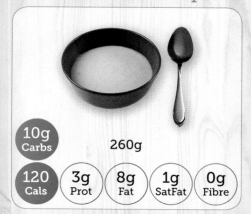

10g Carbs

260g

120 Cals

3g Prot

8g Fat

1g SatFat

0g Fibre

Onion Soup

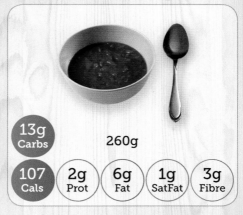

13g Carbs

260g

107 Cals

2g Prot

6g Fat

1g SatFat

3g Fibre

Tomato Soup (cream of)

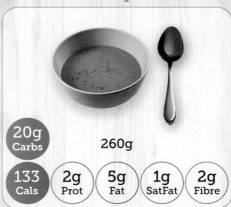

20g Carbs

260g

133 Cals

2g Prot

5g Fat

1g SatFat

2g Fibre

Butter

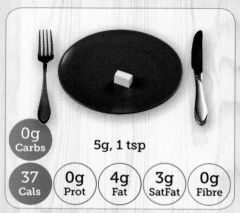

0g
Carbs

5g, 1 tsp

37
Cals

0g
Prot

4g
Fat

3g
SatFat

0g
Fibre

Margarine

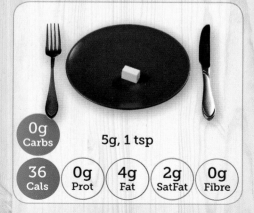

0g
Carbs

5g, 1 tsp

36
Cals

0g
Prot

4g
Fat

2g
SatFat

0g
Fibre

Margarine (light)

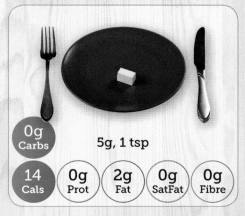

0g Carbs

5g, 1 tsp

14 Cals | 0g Prot | 2g Fat | 0g SatFat | 0g Fibre

Olive Oil Spread

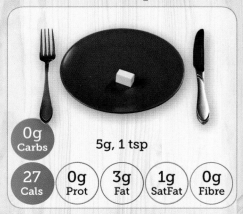

0g Carbs

5g, 1 tsp

27 Cals | 0g Prot | 3g Fat | 1g SatFat | 0g Fibre

Lard

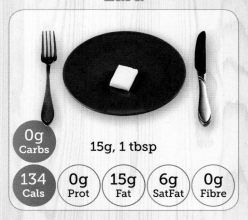

0g Carbs

15g, 1 tbsp

134 Cals

0g Prot

15g Fat

6g SatFat

0g Fibre

Ghee

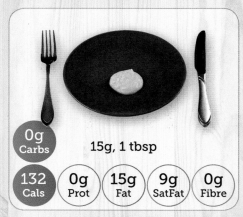

0g Carbs

15g, 1 tbsp

132 Cals

0g Prot

15g Fat

9g SatFat

0g Fibre

Olive / Vegetable / Sesame Oil

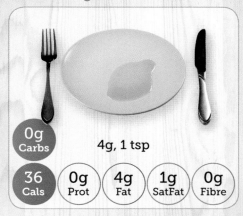

0g Carbs

4g, 1 tsp

36 Cals | 0g Prot | 4g Fat | 1g SatFat | 0g Fibre

Rapeseed Oil

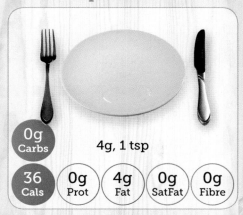

0g Carbs

4g, 1 tsp

36 Cals | 0g Prot | 4g Fat | 0g SatFat | 0g Fibre

Palm Oil

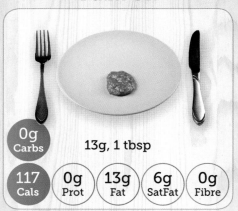

0g
Carbs

13g, 1 tbsp

117
Cals

0g
Prot

13g
Fat

6g
SatFat

0g
Fibre

Chocolate Nut Spread

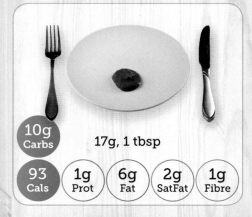

10g
Carbs

17g, 1 tbsp

93
Cals

1g
Prot

6g
Fat

2g
SatFat

1g
Fibre

Honey

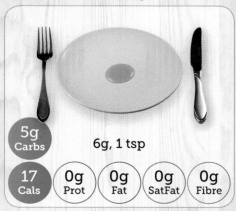

5g
Carbs

6g, 1 tsp

17
Cals

0g
Prot

0g
Fat

0g
SatFat

0g
Fibre

Jam

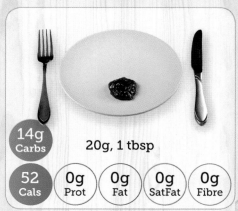

14g
Carbs

20g, 1 tbsp

52
Cals

0g
Prot

0g
Fat

0g
SatFat

0g
Fibre

Lemon Curd

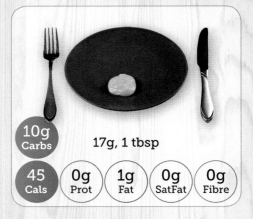

10g Carbs

45 Cals

17g, 1 tbsp

0g Prot | 1g Fat | 0g SatFat | 0g Fibre

Maple Syrup

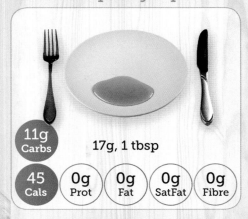

11g Carbs

45 Cals

17g, 1 tbsp

0g Prot | 0g Fat | 0g SatFat | 0g Fibre

Marmalade

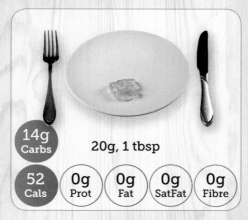

14g Carbs

20g, 1 tbsp

52 Cals

0g Prot

0g Fat

0g SatFat

0g Fibre

Marmite

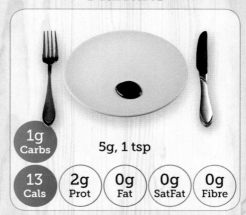

1g Carbs

5g, 1 tsp

13 Cals

2g Prot

0g Fat

0g SatFat

0g Fibre

Peanut Butter (crunchy)

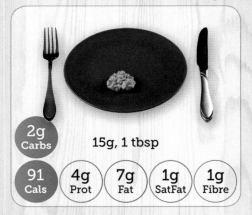

2g Carbs

15g, 1 tbsp

91 Cals | **4g** Prot | **7g** Fat | **1g** SatFat | **1g** Fibre

Peanut Butter (smooth)

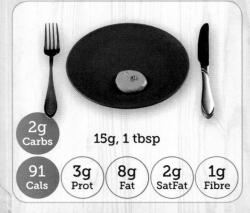

2g Carbs

15g, 1 tbsp

91 Cals | **3g** Prot | **8g** Fat | **2g** SatFat | **1g** Fibre

Sugar (white)

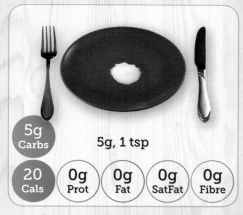

5g Carbs

5g, 1 tsp

20 Cals | 0g Prot | 0g Fat | 0g SatFat | 0g Fibre

Sugar (brown)

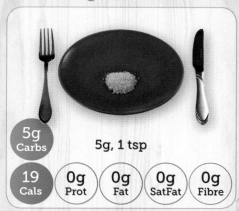

5g Carbs

5g, 1 tsp

19 Cals | 0g Prot | 0g Fat | 0g SatFat | 0g Fibre

Sweetener

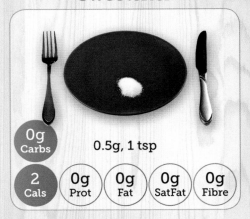

0g Carbs

2 Cals

0.5g, 1 tsp

0g Prot 0g Fat 0g SatFat 0g Fibre

Apple Chutney

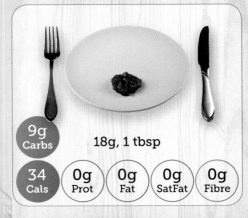

9g Carbs

34 Cals

18g, 1 tbsp

0g Prot 0g Fat 0g SatFat 0g Fibre

BBQ Sauce

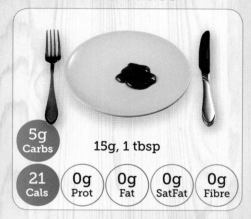

5g Carbs

15g, 1 tbsp

21 Cals | **0g** Prot | **0g** Fat | **0g** SatFat | **0g** Fibre

Béarnaise Sauce

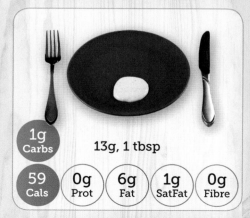

1g Carbs

13g, 1 tbsp

59 Cals | **0g** Prot | **6g** Fat | **1g** SatFat | **0g** Fibre

Brown Sauce

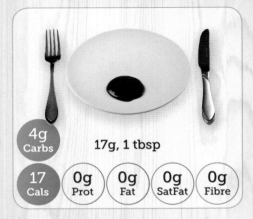

4g Carbs

17g, 1 tbsp

17 Cals | **0g** Prot | **0g** Fat | **0g** SatFat | **0g** Fibre

Caesar Dressing

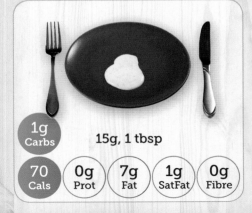

1g Carbs

15g, 1 tbsp

70 Cals | **0g** Prot | **7g** Fat | **1g** SatFat | **0g** Fibre

Chilli Sauce

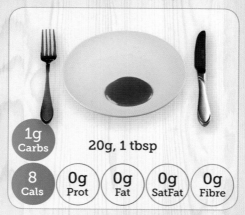

1g Carbs

20g, 1 tbsp

8 Cals | **0g** Prot | **0g** Fat | **0g** SatFat | **0g** Fibre

Cranberry Sauce

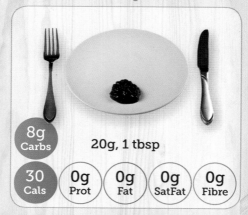

8g Carbs

20g, 1 tbsp

30 Cals | **0g** Prot | **0g** Fat | **0g** SatFat | **0g** Fibre

Gravy

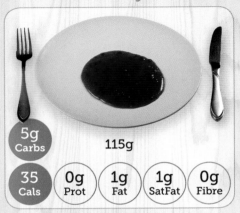

5g Carbs

115g

35 Cals | **0g** Prot | **1g** Fat | **1g** SatFat | **0g** Fibre

Guacamole

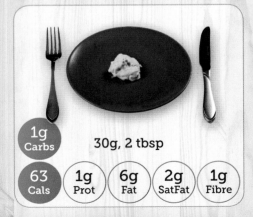

1g Carbs

30g, 2 tbsp

63 Cals | **1g** Prot | **6g** Fat | **2g** SatFat | **1g** Fibre

Hollandaise Sauce

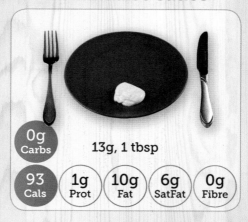

0g Carbs

13g, 1 tbsp

93 Cals | 1g Prot | 10g Fat | 6g SatFat | 0g Fibre

Horseradish Sauce

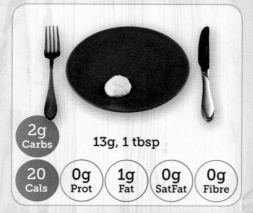

2g Carbs

13g, 1 tbsp

20 Cals | 0g Prot | 1g Fat | 0g SatFat | 0g Fibre

Houmous

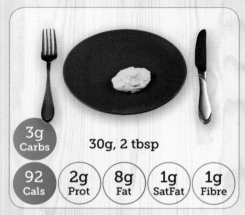

3g Carbs

30g, 2 tbsp

92 Cals | 2g Prot | 8g Fat | 1g SatFat | 1g Fibre

Ketchup

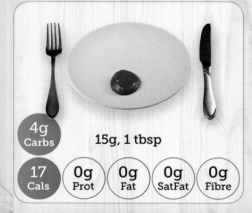

4g Carbs

15g, 1 tbsp

17 Cals | 0g Prot | 0g Fat | 0g SatFat | 0g Fibre

Lime Pickle

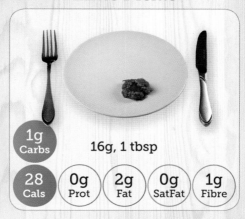

1g Carbs

16g, 1 tbsp

28 Cals | **0g** Prot | **2g** Fat | **0g** SatFat | **1g** Fibre

Mango Chutney

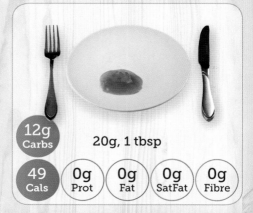

12g Carbs

20g, 1 tbsp

49 Cals | **0g** Prot | **0g** Fat | **0g** SatFat | **0g** Fibre

Mayonnaise

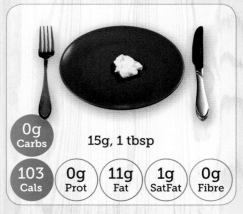

0g
Carbs

15g, 1 tbsp

103
Cals

0g
Prot

11g
Fat

1g
SatFat

0g
Fibre

Mayonnaise (light)

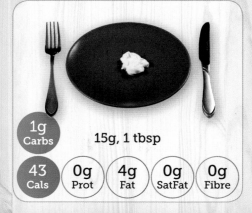

1g
Carbs

15g, 1 tbsp

43
Cals

0g
Prot

4g
Fat

0g
SatFat

0g
Fibre

Mint Sauce

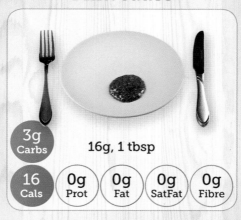

3g Carbs

16g, 1 tbsp

16 Cals   0g Prot   0g Fat   0g SatFat   0g Fibre

Mustard (English)

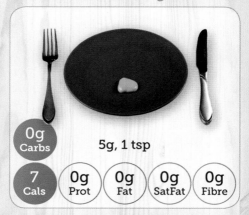

0g Carbs

5g, 1 tsp

7 Cals   0g Prot   0g Fat   0g SatFat   0g Fibre

Mustard (wholegrain)

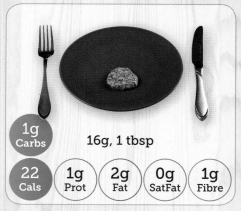

1g Carbs

16g, 1 tbsp

22 Cals | **1g** Prot | **2g** Fat | **0g** SatFat | **1g** Fibre

Parsley Sauce

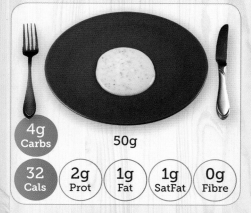

4g Carbs

50g

32 Cals | **2g** Prot | **1g** Fat | **1g** SatFat | **0g** Fibre

Pesto

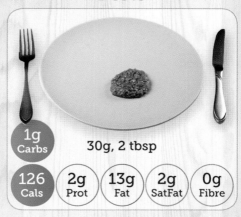

30g, 2 tbsp

1g Carbs

126 Cals

2g Prot

13g Fat

2g SatFat

0g Fibre

Piccalilli

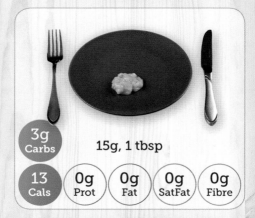

15g, 1 tbsp

3g Carbs

13 Cals

0g Prot

0g Fat

0g SatFat

0g Fibre

Pickle

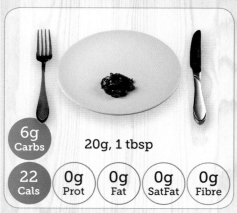

6g Carbs

20g, 1 tbsp

22 Cals

0g Prot

0g Fat

0g SatFat

0g Fibre

Raita

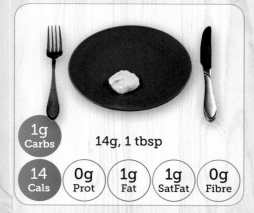

1g Carbs

14g, 1 tbsp

14 Cals

0g Prot

1g Fat

1g SatFat

0g Fibre

Salad Cream

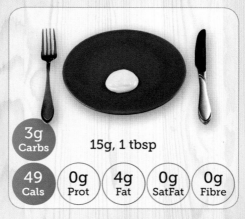

3g Carbs

15g, 1 tbsp

49 Cals   **0g** Prot   **4g** Fat   **0g** SatFat   **0g** Fibre

Soy Sauce

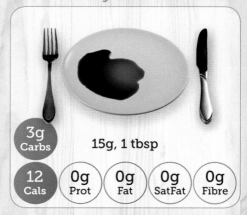

3g Carbs

15g, 1 tbsp

12 Cals   **0g** Prot   **0g** Fat   **0g** SatFat   **0g** Fibre

Sweet Chilli Sauce

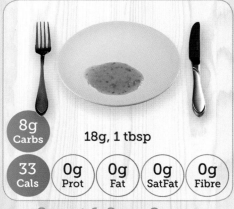

8g Carbs

18g, 1 tbsp

33 Cals | 0g Prot | 0g Fat | 0g SatFat | 0g Fibre

Sweet & Sour Sauce
(takeaway)

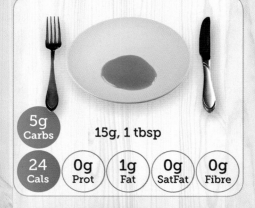

5g Carbs

15g, 1 tbsp

24 Cals | 0g Prot | 1g Fat | 0g SatFat | 0g Fibre

Tartare Sauce

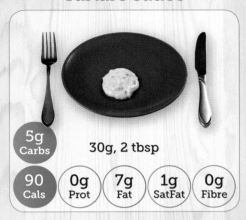

5g Carbs

30g, 2 tbsp

90 Cals | **0g** Prot | **7g** Fat | **1g** SatFat | **0g** Fibre

Thousand Island Dressing

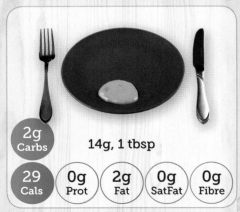

2g Carbs

14g, 1 tbsp

29 Cals | **0g** Prot | **2g** Fat | **0g** SatFat | **0g** Fibre

White Sauce
(made with whole milk)

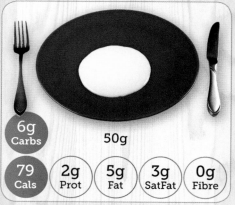

50g

6g Carbs

79 Cals

2g Prot

5g Fat

3g SatFat

0g Fibre

Worcestershire Sauce

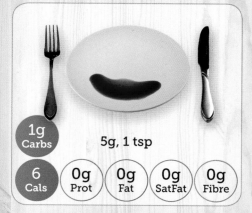

5g, 1 tsp

1g Carbs

6 Cals

0g Prot

0g Fat

0g SatFat

0g Fibre

Ackee (tinned)

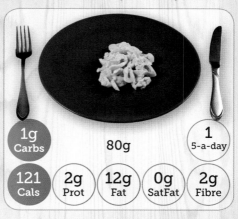

1g Carbs

80g

1 5-a-day

121 Cals

2g Prot

12g Fat

0g SatFat

2g Fibre

Artichokes (tinned)

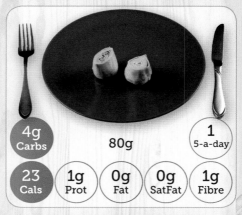

4g Carbs

80g

1 5-a-day

23 Cals

1g Prot

0g Fat

0g SatFat

1g Fibre

Asparagus (boiled)

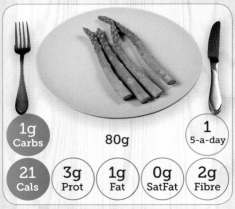

1g Carbs

80g

1 5-a-day

21 Cals

3g Prot

1g Fat

0g SatFat

2g Fibre

Aubergine (fried in oil)

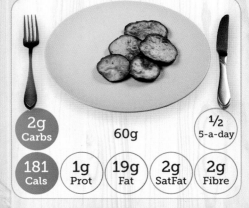

2g Carbs

60g

1/2 5-a-day

181 Cals

1g Prot

19g Fat

2g SatFat

2g Fibre

Avocado

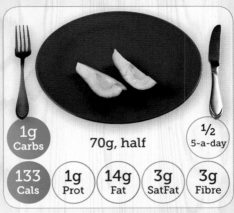

1g Carbs

70g, half

1/2 5-a-day

133 Cals | **1g** Prot | **14g** Fat | **3g** SatFat | **3g** Fibre

Baked Beans
(in tomato sauce)

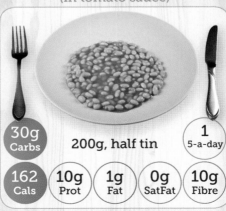

30g Carbs

200g, half tin

1 5-a-day

162 Cals | **10g** Prot | **1g** Fat | **0g** SatFat | **10g** Fibre

Bamboo Shoots

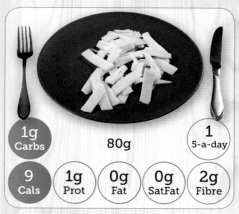

1g Carbs

80g

1 5-a-day

9 Cals

1g Prot

0g Fat

0g SatFat

2g Fibre

Bean Sprouts

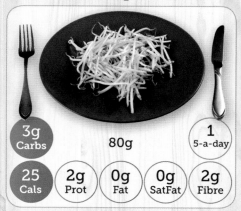

3g Carbs

80g

1 5-a-day

25 Cals

2g Prot

0g Fat

0g SatFat

2g Fibre

Beetroot (boiled)

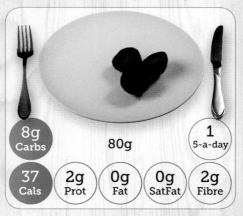

8g Carbs

80g

1 5-a-day

37 Cals

2g Prot

0g Fat

0g SatFat

2g Fibre

Broad Beans (boiled)

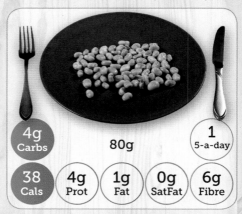

4g Carbs

80g

1 5-a-day

38 Cals

4g Prot

1g Fat

0g SatFat

6g Fibre

Broccoli (boiled)

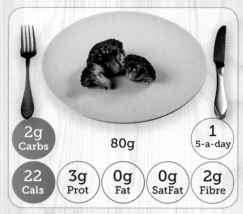

2g Carbs

80g

1 5-a-day

22 Cals | 3g Prot | 0g Fat | 0g SatFat | 2g Fibre

Brussels Sprouts (boiled)

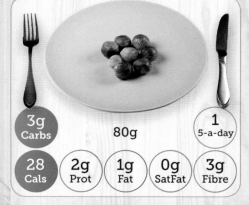

3g Carbs

80g

1 5-a-day

28 Cals | 2g Prot | 1g Fat | 0g SatFat | 3g Fibre

Butter Beans

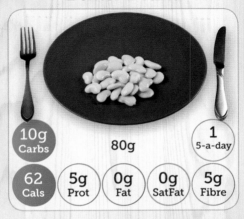

10g Carbs

80g

1 5-a-day

62 Cals

5g Prot

0g Fat

0g SatFat

5g Fibre

Butternut Squash (baked)

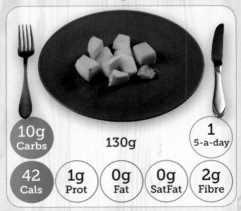

10g Carbs

130g

1 5-a-day

42 Cals

1g Prot

0g Fat

0g SatFat

2g Fibre

Cabbage (boiled)

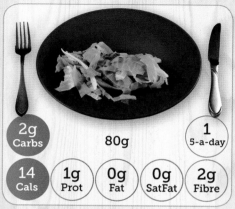

2g Carbs

80g

1 5-a-day

14 Cals | **1g** Prot | **0g** Fat | **0g** SatFat | **2g** Fibre

Carrots (boiled)

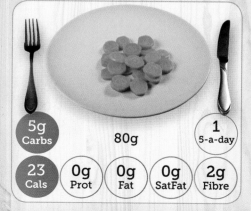

5g Carbs

80g

1 5-a-day

23 Cals | **0g** Prot | **0g** Fat | **0g** SatFat | **2g** Fibre

Cauliflower (boiled)

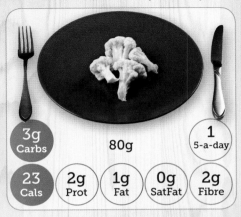

3g Carbs

80g

1 5-a-day

23 Cals

2g Prot

1g Fat

0g SatFat

2g Fibre

Celery

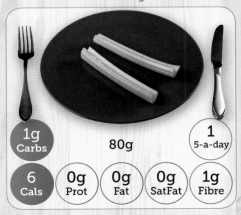

1g Carbs

80g

1 5-a-day

6 Cals

0g Prot

0g Fat

0g SatFat

1g Fibre

Cherry Tomatoes

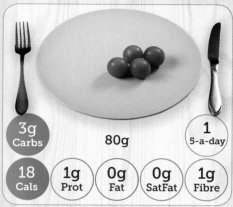

3g Carbs

80g

1 5-a-day

18 Cals

1g Prot

0g Fat

0g SatFat

1g Fibre

Chick Peas (tinned)

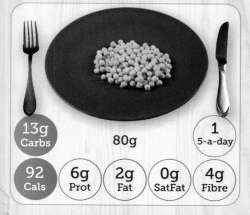

13g Carbs

80g

1 5-a-day

92 Cals

6g Prot

2g Fat

0g SatFat

4g Fibre

Courgette (boiled)

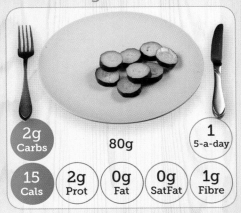

2g Carbs

80g

1 5-a-day

15 Cals

2g Prot

0g Fat

0g SatFat

1g Fibre

Cucumber

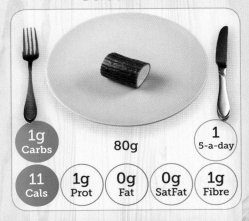

1g Carbs

80g

1 5-a-day

11 Cals

1g Prot

0g Fat

0g SatFat

1g Fibre

Edamame Beans

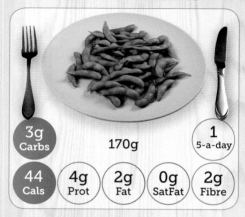

3g Carbs

170g

1 5-a-day

44 Cals

4g Prot

2g Fat

0g SatFat

2g Fibre

Green Beans (boiled)

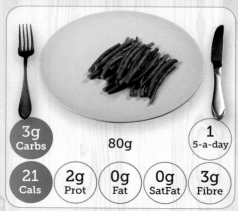

3g Carbs

80g

1 5-a-day

21 Cals

2g Prot

0g Fat

0g SatFat

3g Fibre

Kidney Beans (tinned)

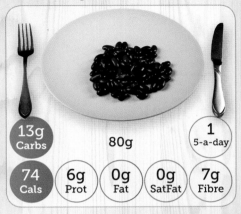

13g Carbs

80g

1 5-a-day

74 Cals

6g Prot

0g Fat

0g SatFat

7g Fibre

Leek (boiled)

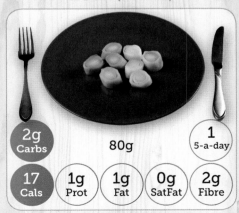

2g Carbs

80g

1 5-a-day

17 Cals

1g Prot

1g Fat

0g SatFat

2g Fibre

Lentils (tinned)

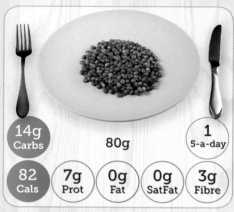

14g
Carbs

80g

1
5-a-day

82
Cals

7g
Prot

0g
Fat

0g
SatFat

3g
Fibre

Lettuce

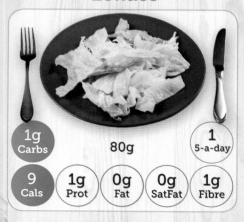

1g
Carbs

80g

1
5-a-day

9
Cals

1g
Prot

0g
Fat

0g
SatFat

1g
Fibre

Mangetout (raw)

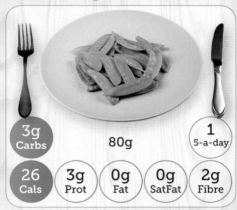

3g Carbs

80g

1 5-a-day

26 Cals

3g Prot

0g Fat

0g SatFat

2g Fibre

Mixed Salad Leaves

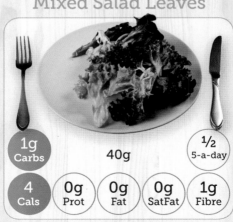

1g Carbs

40g

½ 5-a-day

4 Cals

0g Prot

0g Fat

0g SatFat

1g Fibre

Mushrooms (raw)

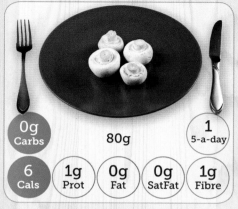

0g Carbs

80g

1 5-a-day

6 Cals · **1g** Prot · **0g** Fat · **0g** SatFat · **1g** Fibre

Mushrooms (fried in butter)

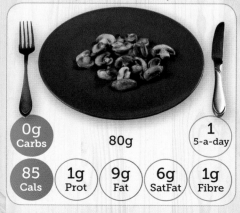

0g Carbs

80g

1 5-a-day

85 Cals · **1g** Prot · **9g** Fat · **6g** SatFat · **1g** Fibre

Onions (raw)

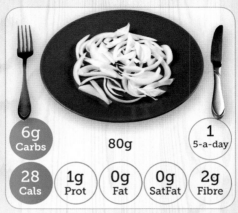

6g Carbs

80g

1 5-a-day

28 Cals

1g Prot

0g Fat

0g SatFat

2g Fibre

Onions (fried in oil)

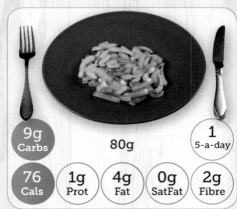

9g Carbs

80g

1 5-a-day

76 Cals

1g Prot

4g Fat

0g SatFat

2g Fibre

Okra (boiled)

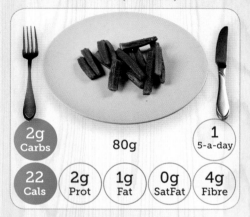

2g Carbs

80g

1 5-a-day

22 Cals | **2g** Prot | **1g** Fat | **0g** SatFat | **4g** Fibre

Pak Choy (boiled)

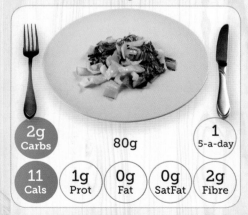

2g Carbs

80g

1 5-a-day

11 Cals | **1g** Prot | **0g** Fat | **0g** SatFat | **2g** Fibre

Peas

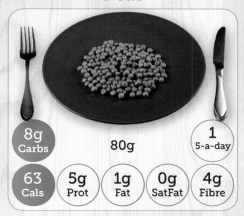

8g Carbs

80g

1 5-a-day

63 Cals

5g Prot

1g Fat

0g SatFat

4g Fibre

Mushy Peas

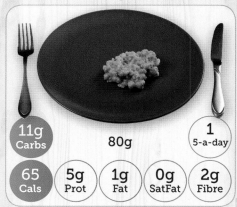

11g Carbs

80g

1 5-a-day

65 Cals

5g Prot

1g Fat

0g SatFat

2g Fibre

Parsnips (roasted)

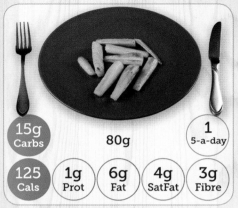

15g Carbs

80g

1 5-a-day

125 Cals | **1g** Prot | **6g** Fat | **4g** SatFat | **3g** Fibre

Peppers (raw)

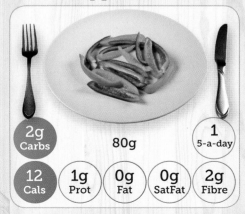

2g Carbs

80g

1 5-a-day

12 Cals | **1g** Prot | **0g** Fat | **0g** SatFat | **2g** Fibre

Plantain (boiled)

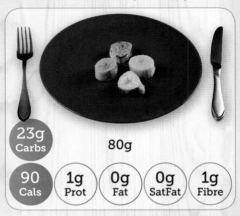

23g Carbs

80g

90 Cals | **1g** Prot | **0g** Fat | **0g** SatFat | **1g** Fibre

Plantain (fried)

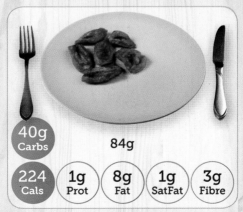

40g Carbs

84g

224 Cals | **1g** Prot | **8g** Fat | **1g** SatFat | **3g** Fibre

Radishes

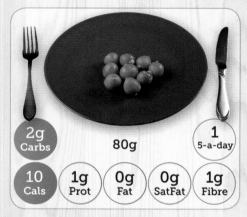

2g
Carbs

80g

1
5-a-day

10
Cals

1g
Prot

0g
Fat

0g
SatFat

1g
Fibre

Rocket

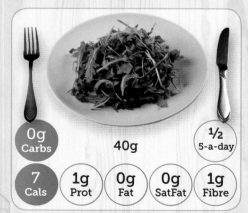

0g
Carbs

40g

½
5-a-day

7
Cals

1g
Prot

0g
Fat

0g
SatFat

1g
Fibre

Spinach (boiled)

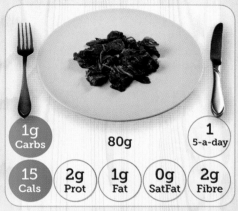

1g Carbs

80g

1 5-a-day

15 Cals | 2g Prot | 1g Fat | 0g SatFat | 2g Fibre

Spring Greens (boiled)

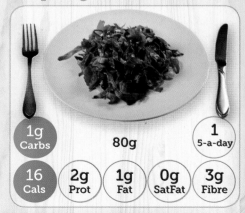

1g Carbs

80g

1 5-a-day

16 Cals | 2g Prot | 1g Fat | 0g SatFat | 3g Fibre

Sweetcorn

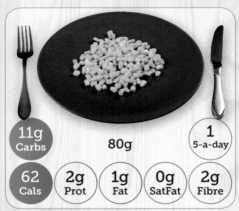

11g Carbs | 80g | 1 5-a-day

62 Cals | 2g Prot | 1g Fat | 0g SatFat | 2g Fibre

Corn on the Cob (boiled)

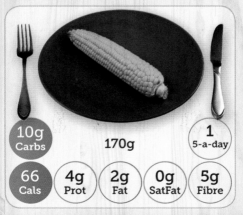

10g Carbs | 170g | 1 5-a-day

66 Cals | 4g Prot | 2g Fat | 0g SatFat | 5g Fibre

Sugar Snap Peas (boiled)

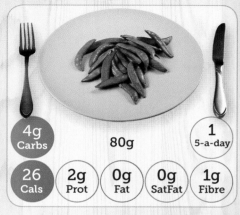

4g Carbs

80g

1 5-a-day

26 Cals | 2g Prot | 0g Fat | 0g SatFat | 1g Fibre

Tomato

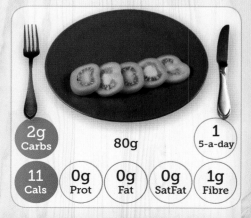

2g Carbs

80g

1 5-a-day

11 Cals | 0g Prot | 0g Fat | 0g SatFat | 1g Fibre

Turnip (boiled)

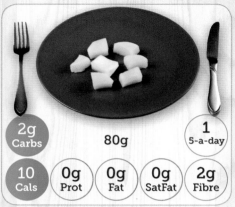

2g Carbs

80g

1 5-a-day

10 Cals

0g Prot

0g Fat

0g SatFat

2g Fibre

Watercress

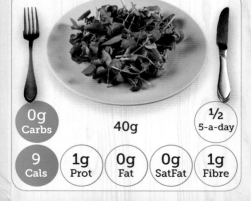

0g Carbs

40g

1/2 5-a-day

9 Cals

1g Prot

0g Fat

0g SatFat

1g Fibre

Tofu (fried)

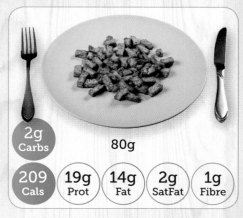

2g Carbs

80g

209 Cals | **19g** Prot | **14g** Fat | **2g** SatFat | **1g** Fibre

Quorn Chicken Pieces

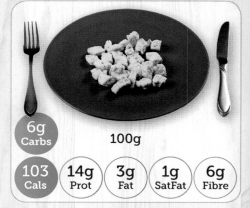

6g Carbs

100g

103 Cals | **14g** Prot | **3g** Fat | **1g** SatFat | **6g** Fibre

Quorn Burger (fried)

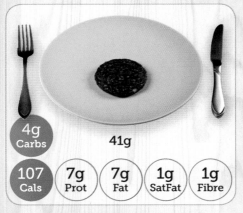

4g Carbs

41g

107 Cals | 7g Prot | 7g Fat | 1g SatFat | 1g Fibre

Quorn Burger (grilled)

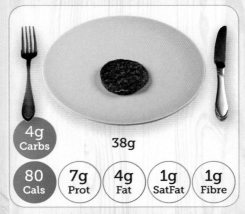

4g Carbs

38g

80 Cals | 7g Prot | 4g Fat | 1g SatFat | 1g Fibre

Quorn Sausage (fried)

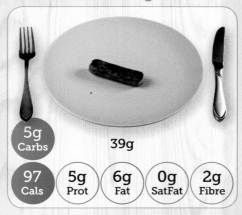

5g Carbs

39g

97 Cals | 5g Prot | 6g Fat | 0g SatFat | 2g Fibre

Quorn Sausage (grilled)

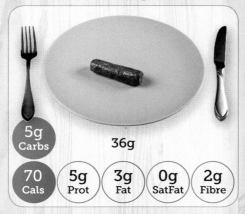

5g Carbs

36g

70 Cals | 5g Prot | 3g Fat | 0g SatFat | 2g Fibre

Veggie Burger (fried)

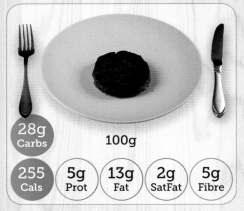

28g Carbs

100g

255 Cals

5g Prot

13g Fat

2g SatFat

5g Fibre

Veggie Burger (grilled)

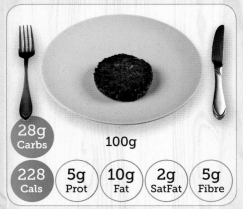

28g Carbs

100g

228 Cals

5g Prot

10g Fat

2g SatFat

5g Fibre

Veggie Sausage (fried)

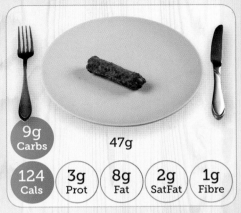

9g Carbs

47g

124 Cals

3g Prot

8g Fat

2g SatFat

1g Fibre

Veggie Sausage (grilled)

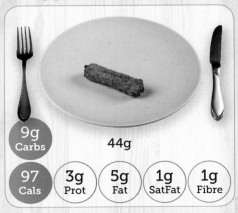

9g Carbs

44g

97 Cals

3g Prot

5g Fat

1g SatFat

1g Fibre

Fruit Yogurt

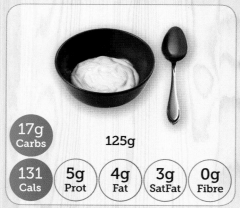

17g Carbs

125g

131 Cals | **5g** Prot | **4g** Fat | **3g** SatFat | **0g** Fibre

Fruit Yogurt (fat free)

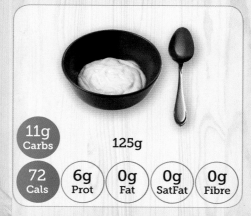

11g Carbs

125g

72 Cals | **6g** Prot | **0g** Fat | **0g** SatFat | **0g** Fibre

Fruit Yogurt Pot

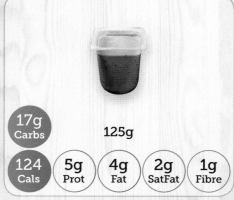

17g Carbs

125g

124 Cals

5g Prot

4g Fat

2g SatFat

1g Fibre

Fruit Yogurt Pot (fat free)

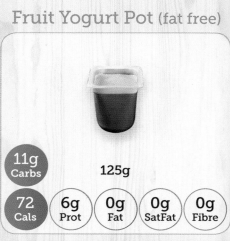

11g Carbs

125g

72 Cals

6g Prot

0g Fat

0g SatFat

0g Fibre

Greek Yogurt (low fat)

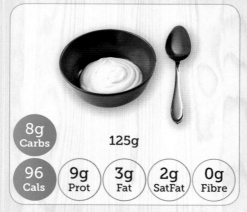

8g Carbs

125g

96 Cals

9g Prot

3g Fat

2g SatFat

0g Fibre

Soya Yogurt

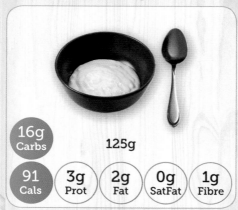

16g Carbs

125g

91 Cals

3g Prot

2g Fat

0g SatFat

1g Fibre

Natural Yogurt

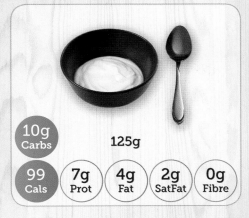

10g Carbs

125g

99 Cals

7g Prot

4g Fat

2g SatFat

0g Fibre

Natural Yogurt (low fat)

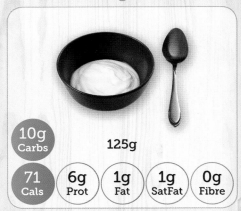

10g Carbs

125g

71 Cals

6g Prot

1g Fat

1g SatFat

0g Fibre

Beef Burger (with cheese)

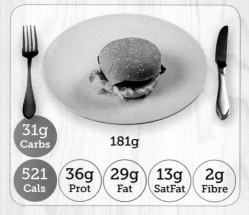

31g Carbs

181g

521 Cals

36g Prot

29g Fat

13g SatFat

2g Fibre

Chicken Burger

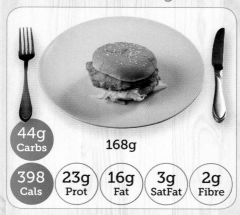

44g Carbs

168g

398 Cals

23g Prot

16g Fat

3g SatFat

2g Fibre

Veggie Burger

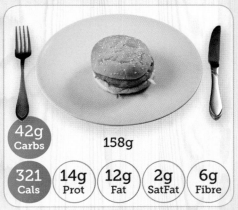

42g Carbs

158g

321 Cals | **14g** Prot | **12g** Fat | **2g** SatFat | **6g** Fibre

French Fries

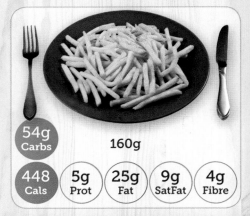

54g Carbs

160g

448 Cals | **5g** Prot | **25g** Fat | **9g** SatFat | **4g** Fibre

Chicken Nuggets

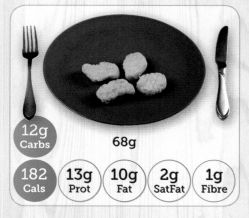

12g Carbs

68g

182 Cals | **13g** Prot | **10g** Fat | **2g** SatFat | **1g** Fibre

Fried Chicken (battered)

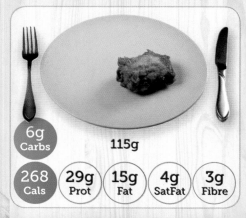

6g Carbs

115g

268 Cals | **29g** Prot | **15g** Fat | **4g** SatFat | **3g** Fibre

Hot Dog

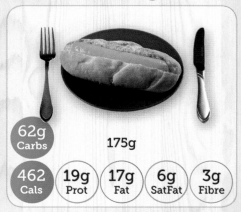

62g Carbs

175g

462 Cals | **19g** Prot | **17g** Fat | **6g** SatFat | **3g** Fibre

Doner Kebab

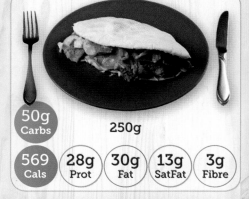

50g Carbs

250g

569 Cals | **28g** Prot | **30g** Fat | **13g** SatFat | **3g** Fibre

Shish Kebab

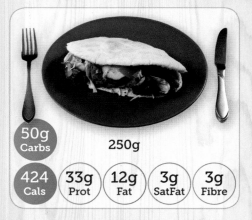

50g Carbs

250g

424 Cals | **33g** Prot | **12g** Fat | **3g** SatFat | **3g** Fibre

Falafel in Pitta

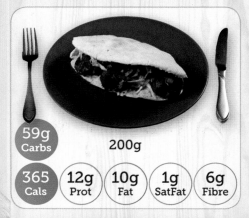

59g Carbs

200g

365 Cals | **12g** Prot | **10g** Fat | **1g** SatFat | **6g** Fibre

Fish

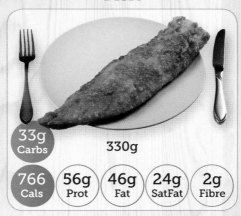

33g Carbs

330g

766 Cals | **56g** Prot | **46g** Fat | **24g** SatFat | **2g** Fibre

Battered Sausage

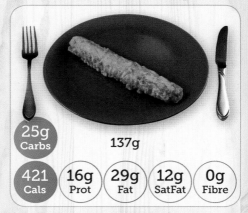

25g Carbs

137g

421 Cals | **16g** Prot | **29g** Fat | **12g** SatFat | **0g** Fibre

Chips

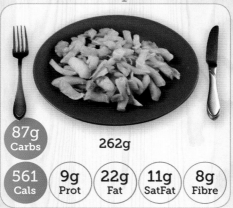

87g Carbs

262g

561 Cals

9g Prot

22g Fat

11g SatFat

8g Fibre

Margherita Pizza
(large, thin crust)

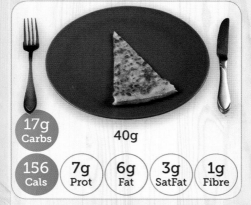

17g Carbs

40g

156 Cals

7g Prot

6g Fat

3g SatFat

1g Fibre

Pepperoni Pizza
(large, thin crust)

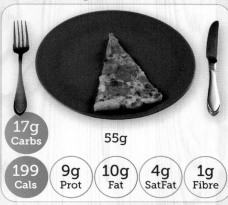

17g Carbs

55g

199 Cals

9g Prot

10g Fat

4g SatFat

1g Fibre

Vegetable Pizza
(large, thin crust)

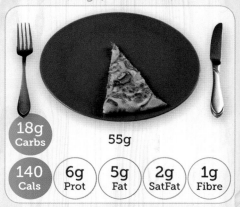

18g Carbs

55g

140 Cals

6g Prot

5g Fat

2g SatFat

1g Fibre

Margherita Pizza
(large, deep pan)

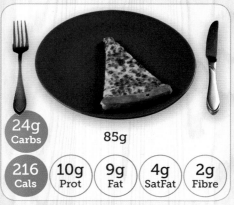

24g Carbs

85g

216 Cals

10g Prot

9g Fat

4g SatFat

2g Fibre

Pepperoni Pizza
(large, deep pan)

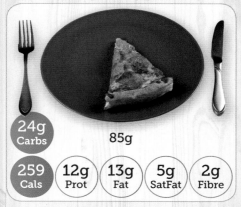

24g Carbs

85g

259 Cals

12g Prot

13g Fat

5g SatFat

2g Fibre

Vegetable Pizza
(large, deep pan)

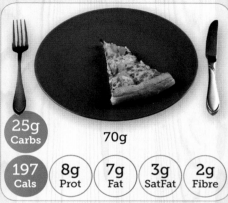

25g Carbs

70g

197 Cals | **8g** Prot | **7g** Fat | **3g** SatFat | **2g** Fibre

Margherita Pizza
(large, stuffed crust)

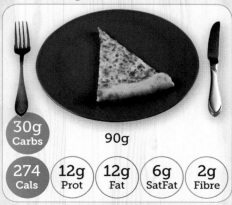

30g Carbs

90g

274 Cals | **12g** Prot | **12g** Fat | **6g** SatFat | **2g** Fibre

Pepperoni Pizza
(large, stuffed crust)

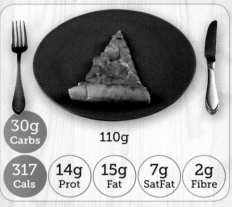

30g Carbs

110g

317 Cals | **14g** Prot | **15g** Fat | **7g** SatFat | **2g** Fibre

Vegetable Pizza
(large, stuffed crust)

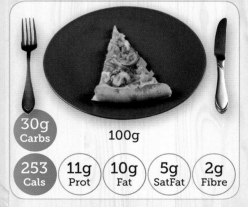

30g Carbs

100g

253 Cals | **11g** Prot | **10g** Fat | **5g** SatFat | **2g** Fibre

Chicken Ball

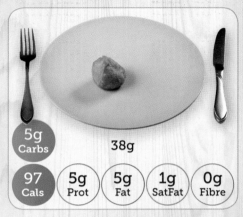

5g Carbs

38g

97 Cals

5g Prot

5g Fat

1g SatFat

0g Fibre

Duck Pancake

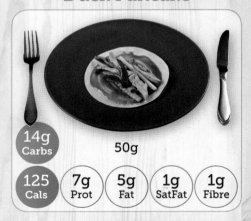

14g Carbs

50g

125 Cals

7g Prot

5g Fat

1g SatFat

1g Fibre

Prawn Crackers

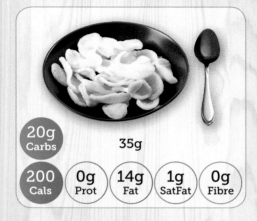

20g Carbs

35g

200 Cals

0g Prot

14g Fat

1g SatFat

0g Fibre

Prawn Toast

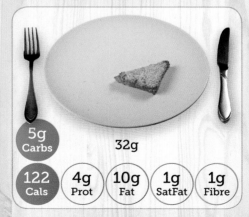

5g Carbs

32g

122 Cals

4g Prot

10g Fat

1g SatFat

1g Fibre

Spare Ribs

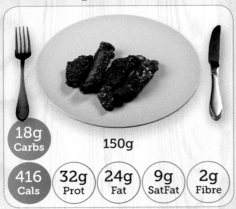

18g Carbs

150g

416 Cals

32g Prot

24g Fat

9g SatFat

2g Fibre

Spring Roll (meat)

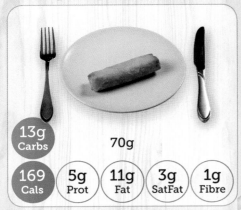

13g Carbs

70g

169 Cals

5g Prot

11g Fat

3g SatFat

1g Fibre

Beef Chow Mein

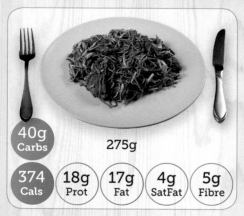

40g Carbs

275g

374 Cals

18g Prot

17g Fat

4g SatFat

5g Fibre

Beef in Black Bean Sauce

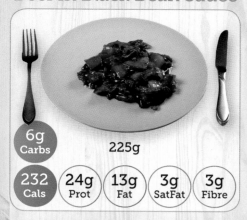

6g Carbs

225g

232 Cals

24g Prot

13g Fat

3g SatFat

3g Fibre

Chicken Curry

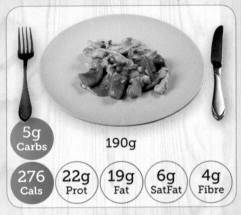

5g Carbs

190g

276 Cals

22g Prot

19g Fat

6g SatFat

4g Fibre

Crispy Shredded Beef

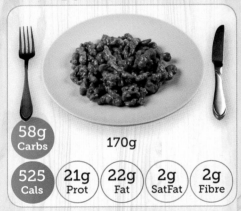

58g Carbs

170g

525 Cals

21g Prot

22g Fat

2g SatFat

2g Fibre

Lemon Chicken

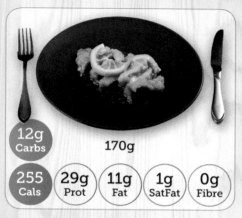

12g
Carbs

170g

255
Cals

29g
Prot

11g
Fat

1g
SatFat

0g
Fibre

Roast Peking Duck

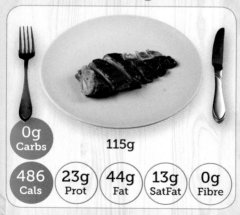

0g
Carbs

115g

486
Cals

23g
Prot

44g
Fat

13g
SatFat

0g
Fibre

Singapore Noodles

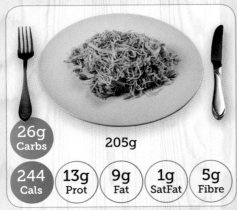

26g Carbs

205g

244 Cals

13g Prot

9g Fat

1g SatFat

5g Fibre

Sweet & Sour Pork

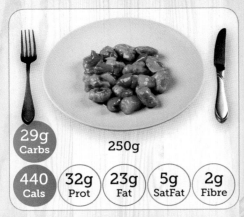

29g Carbs

250g

440 Cals

32g Prot

23g Fat

5g SatFat

2g Fibre

Szechuan Prawns

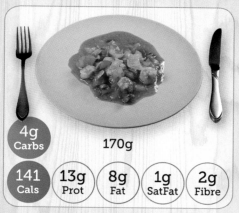

4g Carbs

170g

141 Cals | **13g** Prot | **8g** Fat | **1g** SatFat | **2g** Fibre

Miso Soup

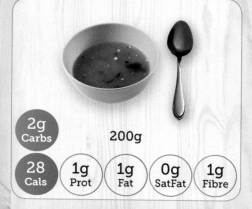

2g Carbs

200g

28 Cals | **1g** Prot | **1g** Fat | **0g** SatFat | **1g** Fibre

Pork Gyoza

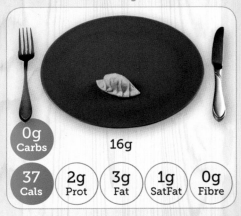

0g
Carbs

16g

37
Cals

2g
Prot

3g
Fat

1g
SatFat

0g
Fibre

Prawn Tempura

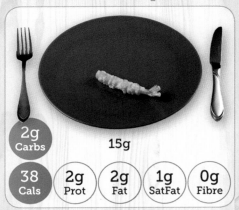

2g
Carbs

15g

38
Cals

2g
Prot

2g
Fat

1g
SatFat

0g
Fibre

California Roll

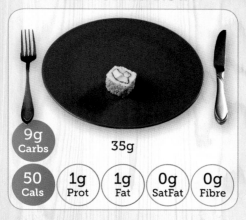

9g Carbs

35g

50 Cals

1g Prot

1g Fat

0g SatFat

0g Fibre

Prawn Maki

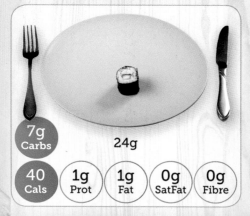

7g Carbs

24g

40 Cals

1g Prot

1g Fat

0g SatFat

0g Fibre

Prawn Nigiri

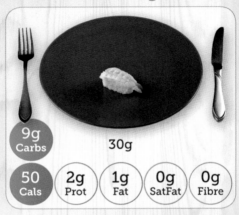

9g Carbs

30g

50 Cals | **2g** Prot | **1g** Fat | **0g** SatFat | **0g** Fibre

Salmon Nigiri

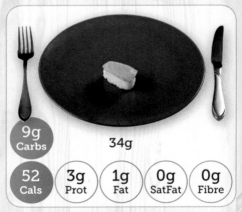

9g Carbs

34g

52 Cals | **3g** Prot | **1g** Fat | **0g** SatFat | **0g** Fibre

Tuna Nigiri

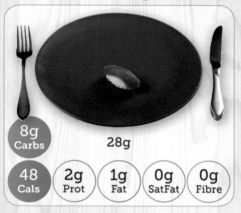

8g Carbs

28g

48 Cals · **2g** Prot · **1g** Fat · **0g** SatFat · **0g** Fibre

Mackerel Sashimi

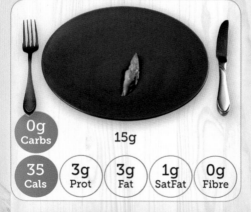

0g Carbs

15g

35 Cals · **3g** Prot · **3g** Fat · **1g** SatFat · **0g** Fibre

Salmon Sashimi

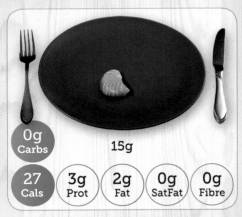

0g
Carbs

15g

27
Cals

3g
Prot

2g
Fat

0g
SatFat

0g
Fibre

Tuna Sashimi

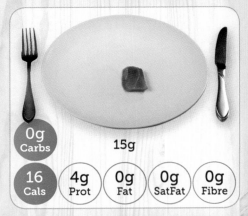

0g
Carbs

15g

16
Cals

4g
Prot

0g
Fat

0g
SatFat

0g
Fibre

Rice Ball

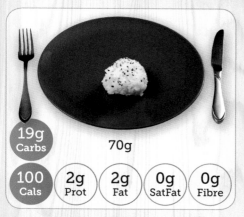

19g Carbs

70g

100 Cals | **2g** Prot | **2g** Fat | **0g** SatFat | **0g** Fibre

Chicken Teriyaki

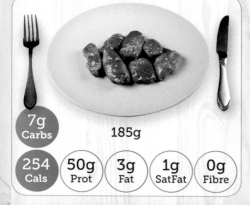

7g Carbs

185g

254 Cals | **50g** Prot | **3g** Fat | **1g** SatFat | **0g** Fibre

Onion Bhaji

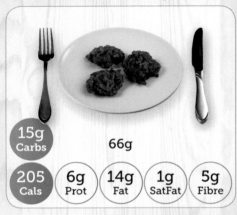

15g Carbs

66g

205 Cals | **6g** Prot | **14g** Fat | **1g** SatFat | **5g** Fibre

Lamb Samosa

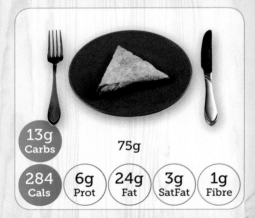

13g Carbs

75g

284 Cals | **6g** Prot | **24g** Fat | **3g** SatFat | **1g** Fibre

Vegetable Samosa

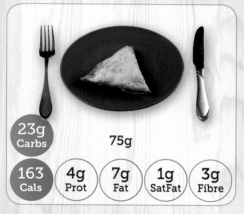

23g Carbs

75g

163 Cals

4g Prot

7g Fat

1g SatFat

3g Fibre

Vegetable Pakora

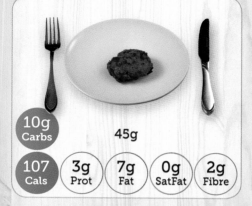

10g Carbs

45g

107 Cals

3g Prot

7g Fat

0g SatFat

2g Fibre

Bombay Potatoes

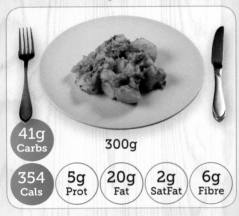

41g Carbs

300g

354 Cals | **5g** Prot | **20g** Fat | **2g** SatFat | **6g** Fibre

Sag Aloo Gobi

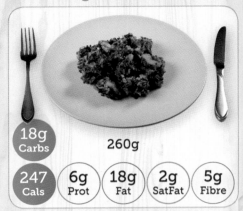

18g Carbs

260g

247 Cals | **6g** Prot | **18g** Fat | **2g** SatFat | **5g** Fibre

Chicken Korma

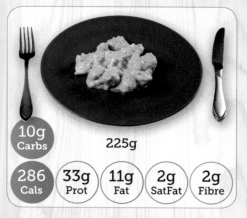

10g Carbs

225g

286 Cals | **33g** Prot | **11g** Fat | **2g** SatFat | **2g** Fibre

Chicken Tandoori

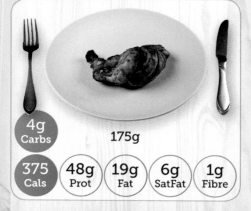

4g Carbs

175g

375 Cals | **48g** Prot | **19g** Fat | **6g** SatFat | **1g** Fibre

Chicken Tikka Masala

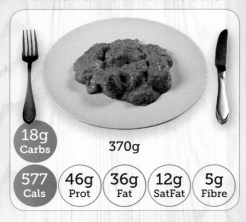

18g Carbs

370g

577 Cals | **46g** Prot | **36g** Fat | **12g** SatFat | **5g** Fibre

King Prawn Bhuna

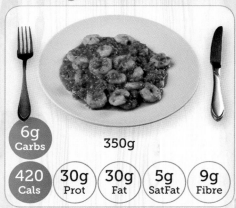

6g Carbs

350g

420 Cals | **30g** Prot | **30g** Fat | **5g** SatFat | **9g** Fibre

Lamb Biryani

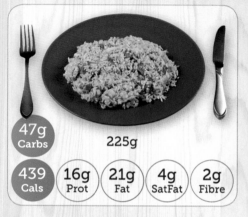

47g Carbs

225g

439 Cals

16g Prot

21g Fat

4g SatFat

2g Fibre

Lamb Rogan Josh

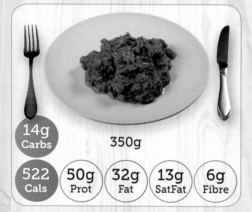

14g Carbs

350g

522 Cals

50g Prot

32g Fat

13g SatFat

6g Fibre

Lentil Curry

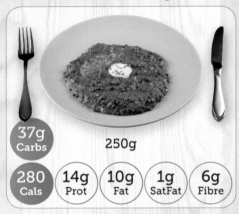

37g
Carbs

250g

280
Cals

14g
Prot

10g
Fat

1g
SatFat

6g
Fibre

Vegetable Curry

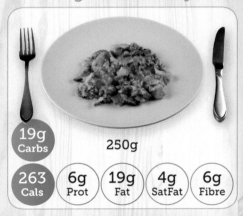

19g
Carbs

250g

263
Cals

6g
Prot

19g
Fat

4g
SatFat

6g
Fibre

Beef Red Curry

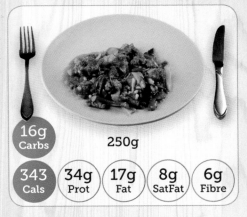

16g Carbs

250g

343 Cals | **34g** Prot | **17g** Fat | **8g** SatFat | **6g** Fibre

Chicken Green Curry

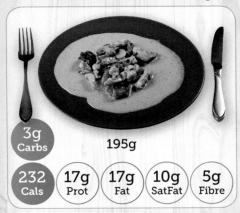

3g Carbs

195g

232 Cals | **17g** Prot | **17g** Fat | **10g** SatFat | **5g** Fibre

Beef Massaman Curry

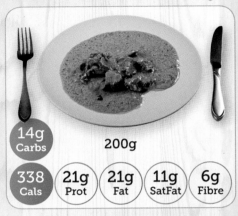

14g Carbs

200g

338 Cals | **21g** Prot | **21g** Fat | **11g** SatFat | **6g** Fibre

Prawn Pad Thai

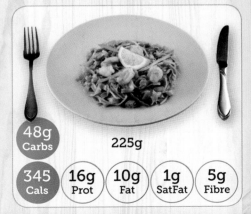

48g Carbs

225g

345 Cals | **16g** Prot | **10g** Fat | **1g** SatFat | **5g** Fibre

Chicken, Prawn & Pineapple Rice

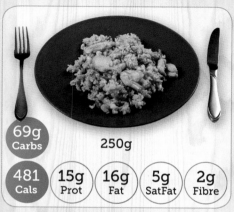

69g Carbs

250g

481 Cals

15g Prot

16g Fat

5g SatFat

2g Fibre

Chicken Satay

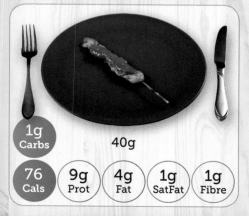

1g Carbs

40g

76 Cals

9g Prot

4g Fat

1g SatFat

1g Fibre

Tom Yum Soup (prawn)

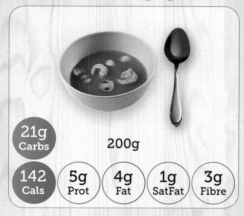

21g Carbs

200g

142 Cals

5g Prot

4g Fat

1g SatFat

3g Fibre

Nasi Goreng

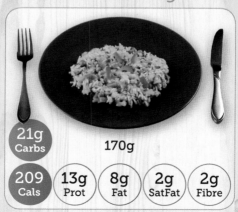

21g Carbs

170g

209 Cals

13g Prot

8g Fat

2g SatFat

2g Fibre

Paella

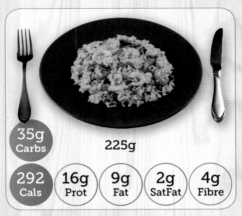

35g Carbs

225g

292 Cals | **16g** Prot | **9g** Fat | **2g** SatFat | **4g** Fibre

Nachos with Cheese

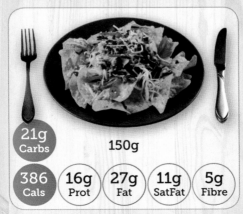

21g Carbs

150g

386 Cals | **16g** Prot | **27g** Fat | **11g** SatFat | **5g** Fibre

Bean Burrito

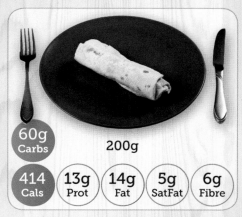

60g Carbs

200g

414 Cals

13g Prot

14g Fat

5g SatFat

6g Fibre

Bean Quesadilla

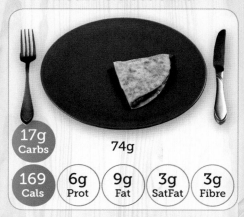

17g Carbs

74g

169 Cals

6g Prot

9g Fat

3g SatFat

3g Fibre

Beef Taco

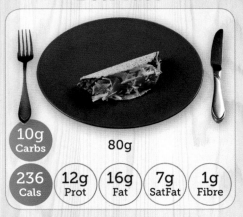

10g Carbs

80g

236 Cals | **12g** Prot | **16g** Fat | **7g** SatFat | **1g** Fibre

Chicken Burrito

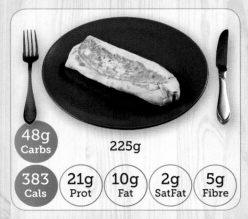

48g Carbs

225g

383 Cals | **21g** Prot | **10g** Fat | **2g** SatFat | **5g** Fibre

Chicken Enchilada

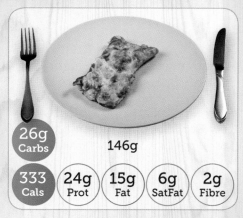

26g
Carbs

146g

333
Cals

24g
Prot

15g
Fat

6g
SatFat

2g
Fibre

Chicken Fajita

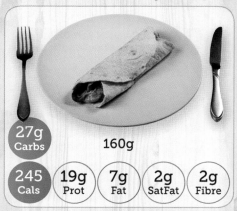

27g
Carbs

160g

245
Cals

19g
Prot

7g
Fat

2g
SatFat

2g
Fibre

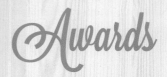

Awards

Carbs & Cals won **Best Dietary Management Initiative** at the Quality in Care Awards 2014

The Carbs & Cals App won **New Product of the Year** in the Complete Nutrition Awards 2012

Carbs & Cals won the BDA Dame Barbara Clayton **Award for Innovation & Excellence** 2011

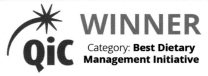

WINNER

QiC

Category: **Best Dietary Management Initiative**

Quality in Care Programme **2014**

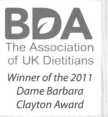

BDA

The Association of UK Dietitians

Winner of the 2011 Dame Barbara Clayton Award

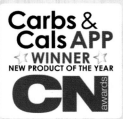

Carbs & Cals APP

WINNER

NEW PRODUCT OF THE YEAR

CN awards